This book is dedicated to my supportive and loving wife, Susan, who wondered if I was ever going to get it written all by myself.

Special thanks to Barbara Dillman for her expert editorial skills in the final preparation of this manuscript and illustrations.

Thanks to Dr. Richard Borgatti for his editorial advice.

I thank all the residents with whom I had the privilege of working in our training program at the University of Western Ontario, London, Canada, in preparation for their oral examinations to obtain their fellowship in orthopaedics. As part of that examination, they had the opportunity to examine a patient and his problem, presenting it to the examiners. This book is the result of working with these residents in preparation for their exam. They are Robert M. Brock, Louis C. Sfreddo, David C. Taylor, William C. Malone, Peter A. Gutmanis, Barry A. McKillop, Thomas W. Phillips, Dennis M. Walker, Roger G. Stewart, James H. Roth, John W. Pepin, George J. Koppert, Thomas R. Merritt, Nathan P. Cohen, Michael G. Rock, Douglas L. Wooley, Robert D. Galpin, Alexander C. McLaren, Arthur A. Schmidt, Paul H. Wright, Ian J. Alexander, Dana A. Fleming, Geoffrey H. Johnston, Garth K. Annisette, Tommy K. Chan, Badie A. Jalaly, Robert P. Landsberg, George K. Aitken, J. Rod Davey, Kevin R. Gurr, Harry Lockstadt, James F. Allen, R. Douglas Armstrong, Robert G. Josefchak, William D. Regan, John S. Halpenny, Moosa Kazim, Graham R. Huckell, Gordon D. Kruger, Anthony Miniaci, Anthony D. Chris, Nancy C. Cullen, Samuel S. Messieh, W. Michael Tew, Annunziato Amendola, Ralph M. Belle, Catherine P. Blokker, Duncan C. MacKinlay, Naresh K. Nayak, Bernard A. Zicat, Nabil M. Sabano, D. Scott Bethune, Robert B. Litchfield, Paul H. Marks, Samuel P. Phillips, Gary W. Stamp, John H. Wood, Mark D. MacLeod, Andrew D. Porter, Nikolaj Wolfson.

An organized approach to
MUSCULOSKELETAL
EXAMINATION
and history taking

Richard J. Hawkins, M.D., F.R.C.S.(C.)
Clinical Professor, Department of Orthopaedics
University of Colorado
Clinical Professor, Department of Orthopaedics
University of Texas, Southwestern Medical School
Orthopaedic Consultant
The Steadman Hawkins Clinic
Vail, Colorado

with 236 illustrations

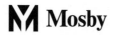 Mosby

St. Louis Baltimore Berlin Boston Carlsbad Chicago
London Madrid Naples New York Philadelphia
Sydney Tokyo Toronto

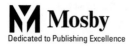

Dedicated to Publishing Excellence

Editor: Robert Hurley
Associate Developmental Editor: Christine Pluta
Project Manager: Linda Clarke
Senior Production Editor: Patricia C. Walter
Designer: Sheilah Barrett, Nancy McDonald
Manufacturing Supervisor: Betty Richmond
Cover art: Sheritt-Krebs Design

Printed in the United States of America
Composition by Graphic World, Inc.
Printing/binding by Malloy Lithographing, Inc.

Mosby–Year Book, Inc.
11830 Westline Industrial Drive
St. Louis, Missouri 63146

Library of Congress Cataloging in Publication Data

Hawkins, Richard J.
   An organized approach to musculoskeletal examination and history taking / Richard J. Hawkins.
        p.   cm.
   Includes bibliographical references and index.
   ISBN 0-8151-4162-9
   1. Musculoskeletal system—Diseases—Diagnosis.
   2. Medical history taking.   3. Physical diagnosis.   I. Title.
   [DNLM: 1. Musculoskeletal Diseases—diagnosis.
   2. Physical Examination—methods.   3. Medical History
   Taking—methods.   WE 141
   H394o 1995]
   RC925.H385   1995
   616.7'075—dc20
   DNLM/DLC
   for Library of Congress   94-28871
                                                                CIP

95 96 97 98 99 / 9 8 7 6 5 4 3 2 1

Preface

This book describes an organized format for examination of the musculoskeletal system, with a prelude to history taking and presentation. Unlike other texts, it does not focus on individual joints or parts, but rather offers the principles that can be applied to any joint or part. It does not include the specifics and special aspects of all physical examination features related to a part, but simply uses different joints as examples to illustrate the format and principles. In this manner it is hoped that the clinician can adopt this or a modified format to approach examination of the musculoskeletal system regardless of part, complaint, or setting.

The successful treatment of any condition relating to the musculoskeletal system requires an accurate diagnosis. To achieve this, all pieces of information pertaining to the patient's complaint need to be collected and analyzed. It is often easy to overlook the most basic clinical skills of history and physical examination, relying instead on high-powered investigative aids. These aids play a role in confirming an established diagnosis or occasionally assist in the challenging presentation. However, in the vast majority of cases, a working diagnosis can be reached following an appropriate history and careful physical examination.

The musculoskeletal system presents a broad spectrum of anatomical structures, undergoing a multitude of pathological processes in a variety of clinical settings. This complexity requires a comprehensive and efficient approach to physical examination. The purpose of the following discussion is to provide a tightly organized format that is universally applicable to each anatomical area and pathological process. Physical examination remains an art, rather than an exact science. Much of the assimilated information of a physical examination is carefully documented with medical charting; however, much more information is observed and noted in the examiner's mind. All of this information is considered to assist in establishing a diagnosis.

Clinical assessment should avoid focusing too quickly on a specific complaint for fear of missing a generalized disorder which might influence diagnosis, treatment, and expectations. Therefore, a general history and general physical examination, at least at a cursory level, is helpful before rushing to examine a specific area. For example, adhesive capsulitis can occur in patients with diabetes, often with a more refractory course; both physician and patient should be aware of this. Similarly, the steroid-dependent patient with rheumatoid arthritis has a high risk of complications following surgery, often related to healing and poor tissue quality.

Hopefully, those who read this book will be challenged to organize their approach to physical examination to be thorough and complete. The history of each patient must proceed through orderly progression to ensure clarity of presentation to our colleagues.

Contents

Chapter

I

Organization of the History

An organized approach to taking a patient's history might follow the format of chief complaint, history of present illness, past medical history, family and social history, review of systems, and a physical examination. The scope of this approach depends on the setting. For example, examining an athlete injured on the football field requires a different approach than examining the same athlete in the doctor's office.

The physician's thought processes must be organized to provide comfort in allowing a systematic approach to both history and physical examination. As a result, the completed documentation in the medical file and communication with colleagues will be clear and will follow a logical pattern.

Before describing a format for examining the musculoskeletal system, several salient techniques in taking a relevant history should be emphasized.

The Interview

The role of taking a history, that is seeking out the pertinent facts, in an orderly fashion cannot be overemphasized. Very often in a patient who presents with complaints about the musculoskeletal system, as with complaints about other systems, the diagnosis is provisionally established in the initial 30 to 60 seconds of the interview.

Two important facts play a major role in leading to a diagnosis: the patient's chief complaint and the patient's age. For example, the most common cause of shoulder pain in a 70-year-old is rotator cuff pathology, whereas the usual cause of knee pain in a 13-year-old is a patellofemoral syndrome. Knowing these two facts often provides a high index of suspicion as to the diagnostic probabilities. In questioning a patient with regard to a clinical problem, two distinct areas are explored: the specific problem related to the part and how this problem interacts with the patient's general health and environment. In addition to the sex of the patient, which is obvious at the inception of the interview, occupation may influence the entire process of history taking. The complaints and resultant diagnosis in a 60-year-old farmer may vary considerably from a 16-year-old high school athlete or a 35-year-old homemaker. In a patient who has a musculoskeletal complaint, all of these features are encompassed in the initial presentation to colleagues.

In addition to the patient's chief complaint, age, sex, and occupation, other features such as marital status, level of participation in sports, leisure-time activities, and any history of trauma may be pivotal. These factors often surface in the subsequent interview, thereby providing an impression of the patient and serving as informal discussion points to help relax the patient, facilitating the remainder of the interview and examination. Early on, the physician should know whether the situation is related to Worker's Compensation or is litigious. These initial facts provide additional understanding of the patient's problems and objectives in seeking medical attention.

Obviously, the examiner must quickly establish a rapport with the patient by behaving in a friendly manner, thereby gaining the patient's confidence and thus allowing retrieval of the necessary information.

The Initial Questions

The physician must carefully consider the patient's emotional state. Sometimes the pain can be overbearing, influencing the emotional state of the patient, frequently to the point of depression. The physician must carefully consider and appreciate such situations. In an athlete with marked pain and swelling who has had a significant knee injury, perhaps fearing the end of his career, emotions run high; eliciting the cooperation of the patient in such circumstances may prove challenging.

At the outset of the interview, the physician must establish the predominant presenting symptom or symptoms, carefully guiding the direction and flow of the interview, although the patient should be allowed time to speak freely. During an interview, it is common for a patient to wander from the current complaint, presenting a rather extended explanation. While a busy medical practice does not allow for wasted time, redirecting the interview must be done in a compassionate and polite manner. The examiner must keep in mind, however, that mistakes are made by physicians not listening, or more important not hearing, when the patient speaks. As in physical examination, the physician must have a clear, organized, and comprehensive approach when taking a patient history. So, even though the interview should be physician-directed, the physician must always remember that listening to the patient is of paramount importance. Achieving both goals truly encompasses the art of medicine.

History Documentation

The history is documented appropriately in medical charting by following the orderly format taught in medical schools:

- presentation or chief complaint
- history of current illness
- other medical history
- family and social history
- review of systems

This should be followed by the appropriate physical examination. At the completion of the history and physical examination, the physician should be able to provide a provisional diagnosis and offer a suggested management program.

The verbal presentation to colleagues of a patient with a musculoskeletal complaint follows an orderly manner; for example, the physician might say the following. This 39-year-old male truck driver presents with a chief complaint of left knee pain. His history dates back four years to his involvement in a motor vehicle accident, striking his knee against the dashboard. Then the presenter should be asked to describe the sequence of events, the progression of the process, the treatments taken and their effects, and the current degree of pain and its related disability. Other features relating to past history, functional inquiry, family history, and medications may be relevant. At this stage, the presenter then proceeds to a description of the physical examination.

Clinical Setting

The emphasis and technique of both history taking and physical examination depends on the clinical setting. An acute versus a chronic complaint, the severity of the problem, and the surrounding environment all influence the scope of the history taking and physical examination. A traumatized, comatose patient presenting in the emergency room is approached differently than the patient who presents in an office environment with a chronically painful hip. In the former circumstance, the history is rapidly assimilated from surrounding personnel and from obvious deductions relating to the presenting situation. Simultaneously, the examiner focuses on the ABCs (airway, bleeding, circulation) related to the trauma setting.

The clinical setting provides the framework for the focus and direction of the history, which in turn influences the subsequent physical examination. The chief complaint leading to a suspected diagnosis often determines the emphasis of the physical examination. For example, on the one hand, the examiner might spend a significant part of the examination on instability assessment in a young adult male who presents with giving way of the knee, whereas on the other, the examiner may spend more time with range of motion in an elderly male who presents with a painful hip.

Chief Complaints or Presenting Symptoms

At the onset of the interview, the physician must establish the predominant presenting symptom or symptoms. Most patients with musculoskeletal problems present with a chief complaint such as ankle pain, a locking or a giving way of the knee, a shoulder popping out of place, neck pain, low back pain, weakness of an arm, or a deformed part such as a crooked finger. Many patients with musculoskeletal problems have a chief complaint of pain, but often they have additional or secondary complaints such as weakness, deformity, or a functional disability. Occasionally, however, patients do not have a chief complaint, rather, they present with a myriad of complaints that are often confusing, sometimes encompassing a generalized systemic disease and sometimes unclear in causation.

The patient may present with a chronic musculoskeletal problem or following an acute injury. With an acute injury, the physician must determine pathology, such as a vascular injury with a dislocated knee, in order to avert any catastrophic problem.

Complex Presenting Symptoms

Sometimes a patient presents with symptoms and complaints relating to different areas in the musculo-skeletal system. These complaints often lead the examiner to appreciate that the patient has an underlying disease process such as rheumatoid arthritis affecting his general well-being. While each complaint requires individual consideration, it should be related to the overall situation.

(

Chapter

2

How to Obtain a History of Current Illness

Onset

Once the primary complaint is established, the physician must endeavor to take the patient back to its onset. The patient may be unclear as to how or why symptoms started and may describe a spontaneous onset. However, onset is often related to work or follows overuse, such as a change in the pattern of activities in the days or weeks preceding symptoms. This may occur with a change in the type of work, for example, excessive use of the arm overhead in an activity such as painting a house. When trauma is responsible, the degree, mechanism, and events surrounding the accident are considered.

The specific events surrounding an acute or traumatic event that relate to the patient's presenting complaint are vital. Often, the examiner does not spend enough time questioning the patient about a significant event that may have occurred some time ago. An understanding of what happened may lead directly to the diagnosis related to the present complaint. Here are two examples. First, an athlete who has a rotational noncontact injury to his knee should be asked certain pertinent questions about the specific insult:

- Did your knee feel like it went out of place?
- Did you feel or hear a snap or pop?
- Were you able to walk and support weight on the knee following the injury; if not, did you feel too much pain or did the knee give way again as it did with the initial insult?
- How rapid was the onset of swelling?

Appropriate answers to these specific questions may suggest the diagnosis of an anterior cruciate ligament tear in the knee. The subject of the second example, the farmer who falls six feet onto his shoulder, should be questioned as follows:

- Did your shoulder come out of its joint?
- Could you move your shoulder after the injury?
- Did you go to the hospital to have x-ray films?
- What was the result of the x-ray examination?
- Did you work the next day?

Specific questions relating to the onset of the patient's problem are required by the examining physician if a diagnosis is to be discovered.

Clinical Course and Influence of Treatment

Once the circumstances surrounding the onset are established, the clinical course of the complaint is determined from its inception to the present. During this period, the effects and timing of any treatments are carefully considered. Any response to treatment, even if only temporary, is important. Each time the patient reports a treatment in the process, the response or result of that treatment must be carefully explored. For example, if an injection was given, the physician should ask about its immediate effect for diagnostic reasons and its lasting effect for therapeutic implications. The effect or result of physiotherapy, medications, and even surgery requires careful analysis.

Treatment modalities or external influences that affect the chief complaint are important in this sequence of events. For example, the physician must know the effect various medications have on a complaint such as pain:

Does the patient require analgesia; if so, does it relieve the pain?

How much analgesia is being taken?

Is antiinflammatory medication being taken; if so, is it helpful?

If an operation was performed in the past, did it eliminate the problem, leave the problem exactly as it was, or create another complaint?

Progression of the Process

Throughout the interview, the examiner must recognize the progression of the disease process both as

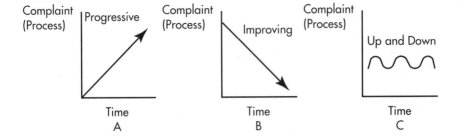

Figure 2-1.
The progress of a patient's complaint process is shown.

appreciated by the patient and as objectively determined by appropriate questioning. Whether the pain is diminishing or worsening might determine the aggressiveness of investigation and influence diagnosis and subsequent management (**Fig. 2-1**). The patient's complaint may be steadily upward in nature, indicating progressive worsening; it may be steadily downward, indicating gradual improvement; it may be a constant and therefore static in progression. It can even run an undulating up-and-down course, sometimes improving, sometimes worsening.

Frequently, when the interviewer learns that the patient who had an acute injury two weeks ago is quickly improving and returning to normal, the interview is cut short and perhaps the physical examination is not as comprehensive as it might otherwise be. Whereas in the patient who presents with a six-week history of progressive, disabling pain with numbness into an extremity, a comprehensive history and thorough physical examination are needed to determine the exact diagnosis, thereby instigating appropriate therapy to potentially rectify the situation. This now brings the physician full circle and back to the presenting complaint of the patient and, importantly, a determination of its degree.

Current Status of Complaint

This sequence of questioning eventually returns the physician and patient to the current status of the presenting symptom. A careful analysis is then made of the many features of the symptom's present character and intensity in addition to the way in which it interferes with the activities of daily living, work, and recreation.

Complex History

Occasionally, a patient presents with a recurrence related to an ongoing problem, such as giving way in a knee that has already had multiple surgeries. The patient may present with a new complaint that may be related to an adjacent pathology, such as shoulder pain in someone who has had a previous operation on the neck. In these circumstances, the chief complaint should be determined; however, the question remains of how far back in the history the physician should go or how combinations of pathologies interrelate. For example, a football player may present with pain and swelling, having twisted his knee three days previously. The recent history begins at the time of the injury three days ago, however, taking the patient back to the original problem (particularly if the knee has surgical scars), which may run a fairly complex course, is often pertinent. The physician must take care in sorting out such a story. Documenting this history on the medical chart and the verbal presentation of this history requires a certain facility on behalf of the presenter or examiner to maintain order and straightforwardness. Eventually during the interview, the physician returns to the true inception. The course and sequencing of events in such circumstances can be confusing and difficult to determine. Both skill and patience are required of the examiner to carefully direct the interview.

Finally, the patient may present with myriad related complaints, such as the patient with rheumatoid arthritis presenting with multiple joint pain, stiffness, and swelling.

Pain as the Chief Complaint

Pain is the most common presenting symptom in the patient with musculoskeletal disease. This is particularly so in the usual office, clinic, or hospital setting. It is also true following an acute injury. The patient's age, along with the onset, nature, and course of the pain, including its periodicity, site, character, radiation, associated symptoms, and aggravating or relieving factors, often lead to the diagnosis. (Periodicity implies whether the pain is constant, episodic with certain movements, or only related to certain activities such as, for example, swimming.) These features will most likely suggest the origin of the pain. In someone who presents with elbow pain, the pain may be due to local musculoskeletal pathology about the elbow or referred to the elbow from somewhere else, such as the cervical spine. Patients are often vague in localizing the specific area of pathology. The patient with primary shoulder pathology, such as supraspinatus tendinitis, often localizes the pain over the deltoid region (see Fig. 3-37, *B*); the patient with pain referred from the cervical spine may localize the pain over the top of the shoulder in the area of the trapezius (see Fig. 3-37, *A*).Rather than pointing to shoulder pain with one finger, patients often use an open hand to describe the location of pain. The *quality* of pain is variable with different pathological presentations. Radicular pain from the cervical spine to the shoulder is often of a lancinating quality, occasionally continuing down the arm in a nerve root distribution pattern with associated paresthesias. The pain of shoulder tendinitis is often diffuse, dull, and aching in nature, and especially troublesome at night.

Pain is a subjective complaint and, as such, eludes objective assessment. The treating physician must, however, gain insight into its intensity and the associated degree of functional limitations. The physician can use several parameters to attempt an objective determination of pain, although many factors influence these parameters. One patient may have a low threshold of pain, and another a high tolerance. For example, many physicians appreciate the high tolerance farmers have for pain and how minimally they allow pain to interfere with work and lifestyle. Nevertheless, the following aspects should be analyzed: presence of night pain; analgesic requirement and its effect; other treatment requirements and their effect; degree of interference with work, recreation, and the activities of daily living; affect on lifestyle and personality; and an estimate on a linear scale by the patient of the amount of pain.

Night Pain

The physician may find elaborating on the nature and extent of night pain helpful. As the intensity of pain increases, it may occur both at rest and at night. At first, the patient may only awaken at night when rolling onto an affected part, but later pain may develop as a constant ache that disturbs, or even prevents, sleep.

Patients may even have to get out of bed during the night, walk about, and rub the affected area in an attempt to ease the pain. Some patients even take a hot shower or attempt to sleep in a sitting position. Consequently, some patients may need sedation for sleep; others may need additional analgesics during the night. Severe night pain is typical in the patient with rotator cuff pathology. Less common conditions, such as infections and tumors, may also present with night pain.

Analgesia

The amount and type of analgesic consumed by the patient provides some appreciation of the degree of pain. The significance and interpretation of analgesic requirements in those with chronic pain syndrome can be confusing. Addiction may occur, thereby compounding the situation. However, in patients with chronic pain, addiction is not as common as previously thought.

Treatment Effects

Many patients undergo extensive treatment for their pain. Physiotherapy modalities such as icing, moist heat, and ultrasound may be helpful for symptomatic relief. Modalities such as a transcutaneous electrical stimulation (TENS) unit or some form of electrical stimulation may offer relief and, if used, suggest significant pain. Prolonged attendance at physiotherapy treatments for pain relief may provide an appreciation of the varying degrees of pain.

Activity Restrictions

Further insight can be gained by questioning patients about any restriction of activities or influence on activities of daily life, work, and recreation. As the degree of irritation and inflammation increases, patients may modify or reduce their activities accordingly. The degree to which patients are able to work or participate in sports is an important measure of degree of pain. Many patients present with pain only related to certain activities, such as participating in sports, which is subdivided into whether the pain interferes with peak performance or actually precludes an athlete from participating. Obviously, the patient who has difficulty with daily activities such as feeding, shaving, and dressing is significantly disabled.

Lifestyle and Personality

Because of severe pain and its emotional effects, some patients may suffer the loss of family ties, the break up of a marriage, or an attempted suicide—all suggesting the ultimate degree or at least the ultimate effect of the pain. Patients or family members may suggest personality changes as a result of pain. These manifestations may be the result of emotional break-down, thus relating the patient's emotional state and degree of pain can be extremely difficult.

Linear Scale Analogue

It is helpful to ask patients to grade the intensity of their pain on a scale of 0 to 10, with 10 being the most severe. This can be estimated verbally. Perhaps the best method is asking the patient to put an X on a line with marks indicating his interpretation of degree of pain, thereby offering at least an attempted objective indication of the amount or intensity of the pain the patient perceives.

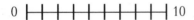

Some people, however, have difficulty conceptualizing pain in terms of a linear scale, while others have a low pain threshold and will overdramatize their pain. Some patients have difficulty answering these questions because of pain variability. The pain may be two or three at rest, but rise to eight or nine with certain activities. These circumstances require clarification. The physician should also formulate a linear pain scale analogue, but perhaps delay this until after the physical examination. A paucity of physical signs might cause the physician to downgrade the degree of pain. The degree of pain, the duration of the complaint, and its course will aid in diagnosis and help direct management. The course, particularly a progressive pattern, can be very distressing.

Degree of Pain or Disability Related to Presenting Complaint

Physicians are frequently guilty of not actively de-termining the degree of severity of the problem as perceived by the patient. This is often evident during general teaching rounds when a junior resident presents a case of a patient who has pain and the consultant is on the spot to direct management. This is followed by a flurry of questions from the consultant back to the junior resident to pinpoint the degree of pain, questions such as does the patient have night pain, how much analgesia is required, does the patient work, and can the patient participate in sports? After securing answers to all the important questions that should have been presented initially, the consultant is then in a better position to suggest directed investigation and possible management. Until the degree of the complaint is ascertained, physicians are handicapped. Nowhere is this more evident than in the discussion on ascertaining the degree of pain a patient experiences and the lengths to which physicians might go and the questions they might ask to arrive at an attempted objective determination of this pain.

Similarly, in a patient who has giving way in the knee, the examiner must determine the degree of disability that this presents to the patient. Many patients with giving way in the knee wear a brace and can participate at a very acceptable level in recreational sports. Others are significantly disabled and cannot participate in sports or may even have difficulty working; all these interrelated features must be determined to arrive at a disability rating.

Instability as the Chief Complaint

Another common complaint heard particularly in an office practice or the clinical setting relates to instability. This is especially true in patients presenting with shoulder, knee, and ankle pathology, and it is particularly prevalent in patients who are athletically active. The spectrum of symptomatology in these patients is broad. In many cases, instability of the shoulder is readily perceived and described by the patient who states "my shoulder often comes out." In others, it may not be so obvious, especially when instability is masked with pain. Patients who have knee instability may complain that their knee gives way with certain maneuvers. Although giving way is a common complaint, some patients have significant apprehension when faced with particular activities in daily living, even when there is only the potential for giving way. Self-imposed limitations may be the result.

The patient may have a history of subluxation or dislocation related to a part of the body, such as shoulder or patella. The patient may have had frequent complaints of giving way, for example, in the ankle. The patient who has had a traumatic insult to normal tissue presents a spectrum of pathology different from that of the patient who has instability related to an atraumatic insult with congenitally loose tissues. Details about the onset often give the most important information that leads to a diagnosis. For example, the patient who falls on the ski slope with a significant twisting injury to the knee, hears a loud snap or pop, and falls upon attempting to stand up, with an additional episode of giving way, very likely has an anterior cruciate ligament tear or at least a major ligament injury to the knee. Another example is the patient who falls, driving the externally rotated and abducted arm in an extended position, and feels the shoulder come out of the joint then pop back in. The patient very likely has a shoulder subluxation or dislocation. All too frequently, physicians do not spend enough time investigating the initial insult, particularly if it is traumatic.

In questioning a patient with shoulder instability, for example, the aim is to ascertain the degree of instability (subluxation, dislocation), its onset (traumatic, atraumatic, overuse), and its direction(s) (anterior, posterior, or multidirectional). Historic features help the physician sort out each segment of this classification relating to shoulder instability. Likewise, patients who have giving way in the ankle almost always have it occur with a plantar flexion inversion stress, in an athletic endeavor, when stepping off a curb, or walking on uneven ground. Patients with giving way in the knee manifest such giving way under varying circumstances; it may occur with deceleration due to an anterior cruciate ligament deficiency or with an external rotation and valgus stress on a planted leg as occurs with medial collateral ligament deficiency of the knee.

Having ascertained all the features of the patient's instability, the final step is to formulate an overview of the disability as it relates to the instability. While the frequency of the instability is important, the ease with which these episodes occur, the mechanism, the ease of reduction, if applicable, and the associated pain and morbidity must be determined. The physician also needs to know if residual symptoms occur between episodes of instability.

Other Symptoms as Chief Complaints

Patients may present with complaints other than pain and instability such as stiffness, weakness, catching or locking, deformity, swelling, paresthesias, or a functional disability such as difficulty walking. Each of these complaints must be carefully analyzed, commencing with the present time and going back to its inception and then following a course of events bringing the patient back to the present. The various features and characteristics of these complaints must be carefully analyzed, tabulated, and objectively documented.

Stiffness

Stiffness of a joint is often associated with pain. Unfortunately, the presence of pain that causes a diminished range of motion can make a diagnosis of underlying pathology difficult. The two types of stiffness that patients present with are, first, an apparent stiff joint and a limited range of motion resulting from pain and, second, true stiffness and a mechanical limitation of motion in the joint. True reduction of motion may be related to either bony or soft tissue restraint. For example, adhesive capsulitis with fibrosis and a contracted capsule can cause a mechanical limitation of shoulder motion. When external rotation is markedly restricted and the patient has a history of injury, a missed or locked posterior dislocation should be considered. Idiopathic adhesive capsulitis, a common cause of a frozen shoulder, often occurs spontaneously in middle-aged women and progresses from pain alone initially, to pain and stiffness, and then to stiffness alone. Its course is usually self-limiting. A family history of diabetes, connective tissue disorder, or vascular disturbances related to sympathetic dystrophy may be related to a stiff shoulder. Other conditions that should be considered are posttraumatic fibrosis or altered bony architecture related to previous fractures. Knowledge of the nature of onset of stiffness, whether it is related to trauma or overuse, and the patient's age, sex, and occupation frequently lead to a diagnosis of underlying pathology.

Weakness

Weakness as a presenting complaint can be confusing, particularly in the presence of pain. True weakness is related to either a neurological or musculotendinous deficiency. The most common cause of isolated shoulder weakness is a rotator cuff deficiency. A history of trauma or a previous painful tendinitis may indicate a cuff tear as being the cause for weakness. With a cuff tear, an associated crunching or crepitation on shoulder movement often occurs, although this can also occur in chronic tendinitis with an intact cuff. Neurological symptoms supported by specific individual muscle weakness or global weakness may suggest a cervical root or a peripheral nerve pattern. Generalized neurological problems such as multiple sclerosis or motor neuron disease also cause weakness.

Catching or Locking

Complaints of catching or pseudolocking occur in knees, shoulders, elbows, and ankles and can be related to intraarticular pathology. While these problems may not be of great concern to some, the high-performance athlete or manual laborer may note significant interference with activities. Associated features of instability may be found with these presentations.

Deformity

Deformity as a primary presenting complaint is unusual, but if present, it is often related to previous trauma, infection, tumors, metabolic bone disease, or degenerative joint disease. Congenital problems such as Sprengel's deformity or pseudoarthrosis of the tibia may be of enough cosmetic concern to the patient to prompt a visit to the physician. Spreading of a surgical scar may be an important clue to collagen deformity, often relating to surgical failure.

Swelling

Swelling often accompanies an acute injury or is present in a chronically painful part. It can be due to an infection or to inflammation, such as a swollen elbow caused by rheumatoid arthritis. Spontaneous, painless swelling is usually due to a tumor, a deformity, or joint lining irritation.

Paresthesias

Paresthesias or tingling down the arm or leg, even into the hand or foot, can occur with neurological pathology accompanying cervical or lumbar root compression. Weakness can result from similar pathology. Paresthesias may be a finding in patients with no underlying neurologic pathology, for example, in multidirectional instability of the shoulder.

Functional Disability

Occasionally, workers or athletes complain that a part does not function properly. For example, baseball pitchers may state that they are losing velocity and accuracy, which may be due to subtle elbow or shoulder instability. A global functional disability may be due to a disease, such as multiple sclerosis.

Presentation of an Acute Injury

The patient presenting with an acute injury poses a different problem than one who presents with a chronic condition. Injuries cause pain associated with a restricted range of motion; for example, the patient who presents with an acute anterior dislocation of the shoulder will support the arm in the "protected position" across the abdomen, demonstrating significant discomfort (**Fig. 2-2**). Associated deformity and swelling may be present. The mechanism of injury and the degree of trauma may be important clues to appreciate the potential amount of soft tissue and bone damage. For example, a twenty-foot fall from a barn roof could produce significant pathology. Similarly, a high-speed motor vehicle accident could produce life-threatening injuries. In acute injuries, knowledge of employment, social circumstance, disability insurance, and possible associated litigation assists in planning treatment and rehabilitation.

Injuries to the musculoskeletal system can vary from a simple muscular strain or contusion to a significant fracture sometimes associated with other complicating features such as a vascular injury. The examining physician possibly can establish a diagnosis directing appropriate treatment and clearly indicate to the patient the expectations and duration of recovery. The physician must emphasize that, in the patient who

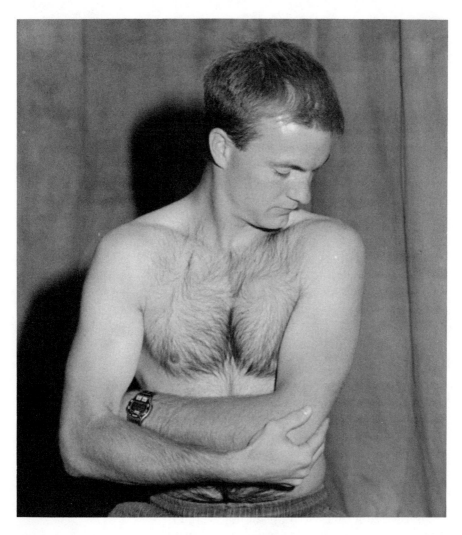

Figure 2-2.
Presentation of an acute shoulder injury is shown where a young patient who has a dislocated shoulder cradles his arm in the protected position (his arm is across his abdomen).

presents with a significant injury to the musculoskeletal system related to an event such as a motor vehicle accident, the most critical determination related to the extremity is the vascular integrity of the limb. This must be quickly gleaned from history and physical examination. Neurological integrity is of secondary importance.

Past History

The past history, although sometimes unrelated to the specific complaint, may be important. During the interview, the examiner might learn that the patient has a complex history of multiple operations. If this is the case, the physician should learn what surgeries the patient has had, such as other orthopedic operations, open-heart surgery, or a hernia repair. Medication such as digoxin and seizure medications are vital to the patient's care. Allergies to medications or other substances may be other important determinations. Patients who have asthma and have been on prednisone for many years could be subjected to significant complications if not appropriately covered with cortisone during and shortly after the operative procedure. Patients who depend on insulin to control diabetes must be carefully monitored. The patient's past history is very important when preparing for surgery because it pertains to potential surgical complications and postoperative care.

Review of Systems

A review of systems is important when assessing the patient's overall medical health. Even though far removed from a chief complaint, the physician should be aware of features such as shortness of breath or the presence of an associated disease process such as insulin-dependent diabetes. These can only be gleaned through specific questioning on a functional inquiry basis.

The physician needs to be aware of medications taken by the patient. The patient who takes digoxin for a heart ailment or antihypertensive medication for high blood pressure or prednisone for asthma could be at risk in a treatment program or surgical procedure if these are not considered. Additionally, medications may indirectly relate to a musculoskeletal complaint.

Family and Social History

A family history of diabetes or malignant hyperthermia are extremely important factors to consider in dealing with patients with musculoskeletal complaints, particularly when operative intervention may be needed. Familial allergies are important in managing patients with musculoskeletal complaints. A social history of heavy alcohol consumption or smoking not only affects the general well-being of a patient but also influences outcome and selection of a treatment program. Occasionally, it relates directly or indirectly to the diagnosis of a musculoskeletal complaint. Indeed, heavy smoking has been demonstrated to relate to nonunions or failure of fusion.

Chapter

3

Physical Examination

General Considerations

The technique of physical examination is both a science and an art, only to be mastered by study and experience. The science is in the objective determination and documentation of positive physical findings. The art is obvious in watching a master physician examine for musculoskeletal complaints. Observing an experienced knee ligament surgeon perform a pivot shift maneuver in the knee demonstrates the "art" (**Fig. 3-1**). Similarly, watching an experienced hip surgeon demonstrate a Thomas test teaches the finer points of examination (**Fig. 3-2**). When physical examination is undertaken conscientiously with this science and art in mind, it produces maximum benefits in leading the physician to the diagnosis and instills confidence in the patient. This examination must be comprehensive and meticulous to avoid overlooking subtle changes that might be important. Experts often state that more mistakes are made in medicine because of not looking rather than for lack of knowledge. While most techniques used in examining the musculoskeletal system are straightforward, others require practice and care in their performance and interpretation. To maximize efficiency and completeness, a systematic approach is necessary.

While the physician may modify certain aspects of the examination to suit the circumstances, the three basic steps in physical assessment remain: look, feel, and move. This chapter expands on this triad, offering an ordered approach to assessing musculoskeletal problems.

Format of Examination

The following format of the examination provides a systematic approach that is universally applicable to various musculoskeletal problems occurring in different anatomical parts of the body. This format can be

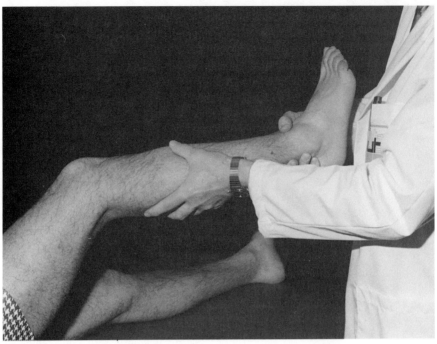

Figure 3-1.
Observing an experienced knee surgeon perform a pivot shift
maneuver for an anterior cruciate deficiency illustrates the
"art" of physical examination.

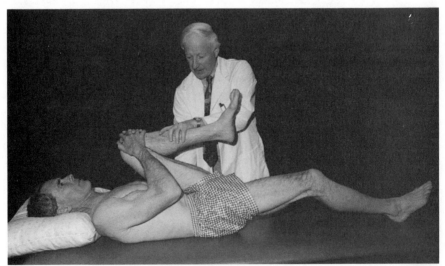

Figure 3-2.
Several years of physical examination experience are required to perform an expert Thomas test of the hip.

applied to the patient who presents with an acute injury; with multiple complaints, perhaps with an underlying systemic disease; or with the usual chief complaint affecting one area of the musculoskeletal system. That is, this format can be applied to a single joint, multisystems, or a specific body area. Even examination of the spine and the hand, although requiring some specialized testing and perhaps a slightly different approach, can follow this same format.

The following format for physical examination is suggested as a guideline:

1. Initial impression
2. Inspection
3. Palpation
4. Range of motion
5. Neurological examination
6. Stability assessment
7. Special tests
8. Measurements
9. Vascularity
10. Gait analysis
11. General assessment

Coordinating the Examination

Although considerable overlap occurs in performing each segment of this approach, for educational purposes each area is addressed separately. While employing each segment, the examiner must coordinate and integrate examination of the joint above and the joint below as well as the joints far afield of the area of complaint, in addition to other generalized aspects of the examination. Examination of a certain part related to a specific pathology may focus only on that part, whereas the overall examination may extend far afield from the focus of pathology. Here are four examples. When examining a problem related to the cervical spine, the physician applies the principles of examination to the spine, to the shoulder, and distally, not only to the upper extremities, but also extending to the lower extremities. When examining knee pain in a 13-year-old child, the hip must be carefully examined; otherwise, a possible pathology of a slipped capital femoral epiphysis causing the knee pain might be missed. Similarly, while examining a patient with rheumatoid arthritis who has elbow pain, at some point the rheumatoid deformities of the hands should be examined (**Fig. 3-3**). If the patient with rheumatoid arthritis having elbow pain must undergo surgery, then a cervical spine examination, including a neurological assessment especially looking for upper motor neuron signs in the lower extremities, will diagnose any cervical spine instability affecting the spinal cord (**Fig. 3-4**). Considering not only the other part but the joints above and below may influence the diagnosis and management of the specific complaint and problem.

When a range of motion examination is performed on the cervical spine, it is appropriate to also do range of motion examination of the shoulder. This is part of the art of the examination, that is, how the various steps in the format are integrated into a comprehensive whole. While examining the patient, the examiner must avoid doubling back and repeatedly having the patient change positions when a more efficient method that inte-

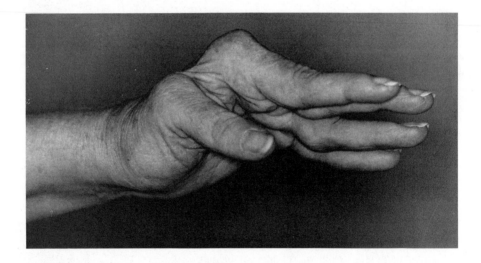

Figure 3-3.
Even though a patient may present with a chief complaint far removed from the hand, if significant rheumatoid deformities such as this are present, they may greatly aid in the physician's understanding of the disease and at some point require examination and documentation.

grates the parts of the examination can be used. While flexing the knee to assess knee flexion, assessing rotation of the hip at the same time is logical, which if painless and normal most likely excludes hip pathology (Fig. 3-5). This would be relevant in a 13-year-old overweight male with knee pain.

Some primary areas of pathology can be located far from the area of the chief complaint. The patient with

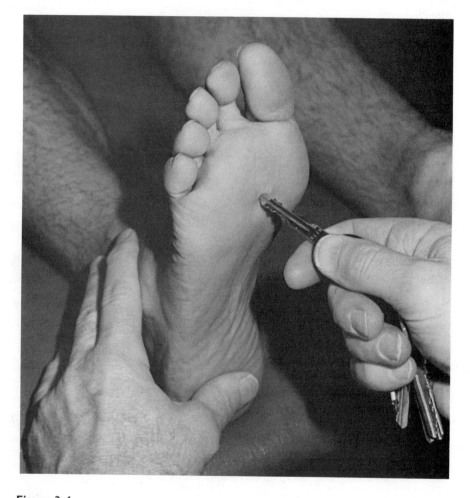

Figure 3-4.
In the patient who has rheumatoid arthritis who is about to undergo elbow surgery, the physician must look for upper motor neuron signs in the lower extremities, such as the presence of an upgoing toe.

rheumatoid arthritis and complaints of leg weakness due to upper motor neuron involvement in the lower extremities may have cervical spine instability. Similarly, the patient with weakness of dorsiflexion of the ankle may have fifth lumbar (L5) root involvement from a herniated lumbar disc.

Applying this format avoids glossing over subtle pathology that may occur. Integrating the steps of this approach by examining associated parts relating to the complaints avoids missing pertinent physical findings that help establish the diagnosis.

The direction and style in applying this format to physical examination is tempered by the manner in which the patient presents, whether in the doctor's office, in a clinic, in a hospital, or in an emergency room. It may also be tempered by the style of the examining physician or therapist.

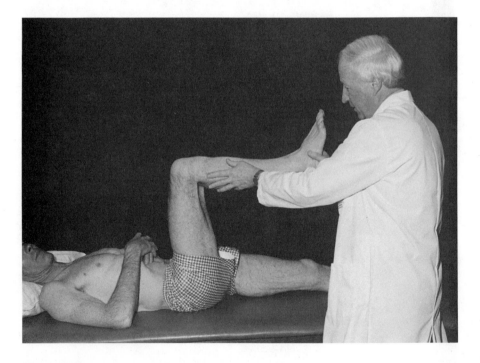

Figure 3-5.
While flexing the knee to assess knee flexion in a patient who has a chief complaint of knee pain, assessing rotation of the hip at that point is logical. If hip rotation is painless and normal, hip pathology is unlikely.

Focus of the Examination

The aspect of this format that receives emphasis is dependent on the patient's complaint and the potential pathology that may be present. An 18-year-old male with an anterior cruciate deficient knee and a complaint of it giving way alerts the examiner to focus primarily on stability assessment. In a 65-year-old male with hip pain and osteoarthritis, the examiner focuses on the range of motion of the hip, with particular emphasis on any deformities that may be present. Then, too, examination of a newborn's hips might focus on stability rather than range of motion. To be comprehensive, however, each area in the format requires some attention.

The bilateral aspects of the appendicular skeleton often permit comparison of the involved and uninvolved segments. Determining positive physical signs may depend on comparison with a normal segment. In the presence of bilateral disease, comparison is still possible; however, objective determination of any abnormalities may then be established by an appreciation of comparative norms. For example, a patient with shoulder pain has 145 degrees of elevation on one side, which can be compared with normal elevation of 180 degrees on the opposite side (Fig. 3-6). Determining subtle thigh wasting associated with a medial meniscal tear without visually inspecting and comparing the wasted thigh with the opposite one is almost impossible. Similarly, describing a limitation of external rotation of the shoulder to 30 degrees without noting that the opposite normal extremity externally rotates to 45 degrees is inappropriate (Fig. 3-7). One of the rules applied to manual muscle testing before a grade can be applied is to compare it with the opposite extremity, which includes many aspects of neurological examination such as sensory, strength, and reflex testing.

Because of its midline location and lack of bilaterality, the axial skeleton necessitates special consideration, yet comparison on each side of the midline is still performed. In the patient with scoliosis, a rib hump on one side can be quantified by comparing it with the opposite side.

The approach provided can be applied to the entire musculoskeletal system, to a joint, or to a body part, allowing modifications to the clinician's specific objec-

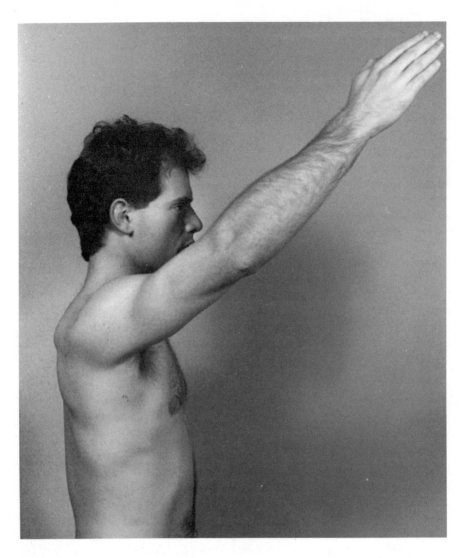

Figure 3-6.
The patient demonstrates 145 degrees of active forward elevation of the shoulder. The documented angle is the arm and thorax.

tives and the patient's problems. The simplest application of this format occurs when examining a joint such as a knee, a hip, or a shoulder. Including a neurological examination as part of the format allows the physician to consider anatomy other than joints in the examination. Pathology that occurs between two joints, such as a tumor in the thigh, allows a similar approach. Although herein many of these features are examined simultaneously with some overlap for teaching purposes, each part is also discussed individually.

Special Considerations

Because of their multiple joints and specialized function, the hand and the spine are unique and necessitate special consideration. Yet even here the described format can be followed, while appreciating that many more segmented parts are present and that specialized testing is required.

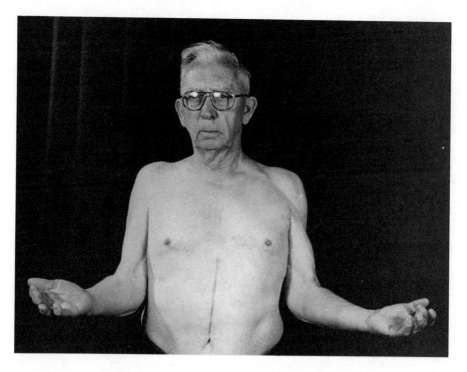

Figure 3-7.
The patient demonstrates 30 degrees of active external rotation with the right arm of the painful right shoulder and 45 degrees of rotation with the left arm of the nonpainful left shoulder. Although documenting 0 to 30 degrees and 0 to 45 degrees on the chart is appropriate, in verbal presentation suggesting that the involved arm lacks 15 degrees of active external rotation is appropriate.

Initial Impression

The initial observation or impression made on first contact with the patient can be divided into static and dynamic phases. The initial impression varies and is influenced by the setting in which the patient presents, whether on the football field, the emergency room, a hospital bed, or in a doctor's office. This aspect of the examination has a significant impact on the focus and direction of the physical examination. The introduction to the patient and the first impressions that result are not always documented scientifically, but are more subjective, with the physician relying on skills relating to the art of examination. Strong forces are present that examiners consider relating to aspects such as dress and hygiene. On first contact with the patient, the examiner obviously formulates an opinion that may temper the relationship with the patient and influence the tone of the examination.

Static Factors

A still photographic impression on first meeting the patient might reflect the following static factors: age, general distress, specific distress, body habitus, and systemic diseases.

Stated Age

On initial observation, the examiner formulates an opinion as to whether the patient's appearance is in keeping with the age stated (Fig. 3-8).

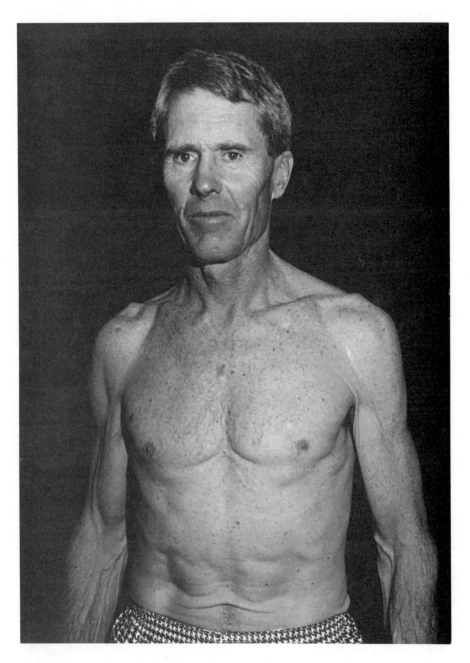

Figure 3-8.
A healthy, active 68-year-old male, appearing younger than his stated age and demonstrating an ectomorphic body habitus, fairly muscular in nature.

General Distress

The degree of distress may be great, as in the patient who presents to the emergency room following a motor vehicle accident and who is in significant generalized distress relating to respiratory compromise or even hemodynamic shock. The degree of distress may be small. For example, a patient who presents with hip pain and who is being considered for a total hip arthroplasty must be observed to determine whether symptoms relating to shortness of breath are present.

Specific Distress

The degree of distress might reveal someone with a dislocated shoulder clutching his arm and holding it in the protected position across the abdomen and chest (see Fig. 2-2). The patient with significant pain in the lower extremity might walk with an antalgic gait or even refuse to bear weight due to this pain.

Body Habitus

Generalized body habitus can be ectomorphic, endomorphic, or mesomorphic (Fig. 3-8). An obese patient poses many problems relating to both diagnosis and management. Conversely, general emaciation of the patient suggests an underlying disease, for example, cancer or acquired immunodeficiency syndrome (AIDS).

Systemic Disease

On initial observation, the examiner may notice that the patient has the many stigmata of rheumatoid arthritis (Fig. 3-3). Similarly, another form of generalized disease may exist, such as neurofibromatosis. Generalized illnesses such as liver disease may be manifest in the form of jaundice. While these systemic diseases may not be related to the patient's specific musculoskeletal complaint, they are often readily apparent and often very meaningful.

Dynamic Factors

Dynamic or moving features relate to the patient's interaction with his environment, permitting an appreciation of the presence and degree of functional impairment and/or pain.

Usually, at this point in the examination, the history is initiated and, concomitantly, the physical examination is begun. Not only does the setting in which the patient presents influence the format, but so, too, do the interview and the responses to the questions in the history.

Observing dynamic factors begins with an introduction to the patient usually by shaking hands. Even this step might provide an indication of some functional disability. Commencing with the introduction to the patient, the following dynamic factors are observed: general disability, gait, specific disability, and functional assessment.

General Disability

As the patient stands, moves, and walks, the examiner should note if any generalized problems such as exertional dyspnea occur with these activities.

Gait

Although formal gait analysis is reserved until the end of the examination, a preliminary cursory assessment of the gait pattern is performed (Fig. 3-9). The physician needs to know whether the patient has any joint deformities, muscle weakness as a result of neurological deficiencies, or leg length discrepancies before doing a formal gait analysis. All these aspects have yet to be determined, suggesting the appropriateness of leaving a formal gait analysis until the end of the examination. Sometimes, however, the examiner immediately notices that a patient has a bilateral Trendelenburg gait, or an obvious limp with an antalgic gait due to a painful lower extremity. The presence of aids, such as a prosthesis, brace, cane, crutch, wheelchair, or even a stretcher suggests the degree of functional impairment.

Specific Disability

A patient who has had an acute knee injury, during a football game may refuse to bear any weight on the extremity or if he does will reveal a very painful gait, and this is, therefore, a significant and specific disability related to the knee. Similarly, if a patient's arm is fractured, attempting to move it may reveal significant pain with marked protection of the extremity. These features provide an idea as to the patient's degree of disability and intensity of pain.

Functional Assessment

A functional assessment of the patient is ongoing throughout the examination. The physician observes how the patient shakes hands or rises from a chair, and even the manner in which the patient with an upper extremity problem removes a coat or shirt can be revealing. The physician should carefully analyze how the patient takes off his shoes and socks, particularly in the presence of lower extremity complaints. The ease

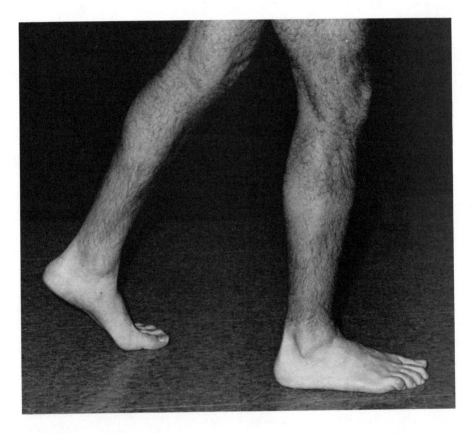

Figure 3-9.
Although formal gait analysis is reserved until the end of the examination, a cursory assessment of the gait pattern is performed at the beginning of the examination.

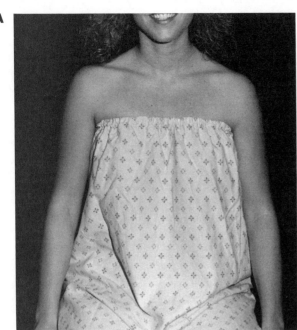

Figure 3-10.
A, B, An appropriate gown for a female patient allows visual inspection of the entire shoulder girdle and upper extremities. The physician must be allowed clear visual inspection of the affected part and the opposite normal part for comparative purposes.

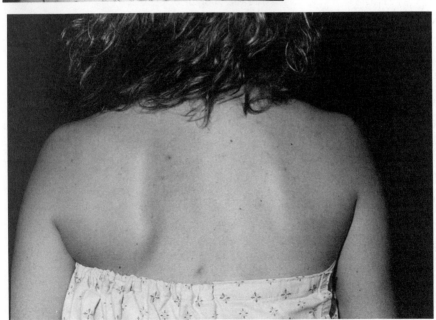

or difficulty with which the patient moves onto the examining table provides yet another element of functional assessment and thus some idea as to the degree of the problem. Although few aspects of the initial impression part of the examination are documented on the chart, this remains an important segment of the examination that influences the direction of the remainder of the approach to the physical examination.

Appropriate Garb

Prior to proceeding to the formal sequence of the examination, the patient must be appropriately garbed and placed in a setting that will optimize comfort and efficiency for examination. The examiner must visually inspect the opposite joint for comparative purposes and, where possible, visually inspect the joints above and below. The patient's modesty must be protected while ensuring sufficient exposure. In the female patient with shoulder pain, an appropriate gown to visually inspect both shoulders is very helpful (**Fig. 3-10, A, B**). In a male patient, removal of the shirt for visual inspection of an upper extremity complaint is usually sufficient. While examining the knee of a female, placing a sheet longitudinal between the legs to cover the perineum provides the patient with comfort and modesty and often aids in the patient's confidence to provide a more relaxed atmosphere (**Fig. 3-11, A, B**).

The usual hospital gowns that open at the back are awkward, particularly for examining the shoulder area; therefore, the examiner should have an appropriate gown on hand for examining the shoulder and upper extremities. In an athletic clinic setting, patients often arrive in shorts, which is helpful for examination of the lower extremities, or in tank tops, which expose the shoulder and upper extremities. The examiner must establish rapport, particularly if patient and physician are of opposite gender, to avoid embarrassment for the patient relating to visual inspection of certain parts. Again, certain techniques can immediately put a female patient at ease, such as placing a longitudinal sheet between the legs, thereby covering the perineum (**Fig. 3-11, A, B**). In moving a patient from a supine to a sitting or standing position, every effort should be made to protect the patient's modesty even if the procedure

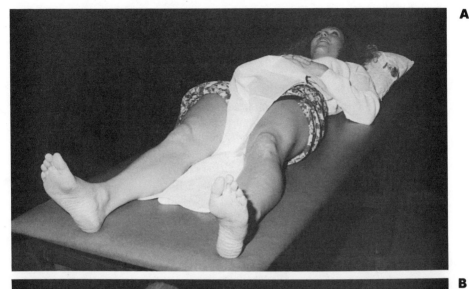

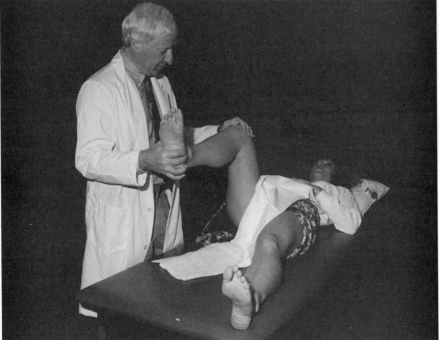

Figure 3-11.
A, B, A sheet positioned between the legs of a female patient
protects the patient's modesty, provides relaxation, and
allows an appropriate examination. A pillow under the head
offers comfort.

must be modified.

During physical examination, the examining room should be appropriately organized and equipped. The examining table is best situated in the middle of the room so that the examiner can move from side to side as required. If the table is against the wall, however, the examiner should examine the side of pathology away from the wall, which sometimes requires having the patient reverse his position. A pillow under the head for the patient's comfort is an obvious requirement to aid in relaxation (**Fig. 3-11, A**). The presence of a low stool is helpful, both for the examiner to be comfortable and to aid in examining the patient if the need arises for examination in a sitting position. To examine patients while seated, the stool should not have a back.

Position of Patient During Examination

The position in which the patient should be examined depends on many factors relating to complaint and condition; the patient may be examined standing, sitting, supine, or in a combination of these positions. For example, the majority of an examination for range of motion with hip pathology is performed supine, whereas most of a range-of-motion examination for the shoulder is performed sitting, sometimes standing, and occasionally supine. At the commencement of the physical examination, the examiner should observe the patient standing, walking, and moving before proceeding to the sitting or supine position. This often reveals the degree of disability and/or pain. Even in an upper extremity complaint, the patient should initially be examined standing. In a lower extremity complaint, several features may vary from a standing to a supine position, such as alignment, muscle contour, and deformities.

Not all patients should be asked to stand and walk at the beginning of the physical examination, such as those who have such pain that they cannot do so. This may also occur in the case of a traumatized patient presenting to the emergency department following a motor vehicle accident.

During the walking and standing stage, certain provocative tests can be performed. In a patient who complains of back and leg pain, heel and toe walking can test muscle strength and coordination.

Inspection

Visual inspection related to a musculoskeletal problem is frequently too limited, for when executed correctly it can provide extensive information that serves as the foundation for the remainder of the examination. The examiner must have a systematic approach to the problem area, consisting of simultaneously comparing contralateral segments as well as assessing the joints above and below and even joints in other areas of the body. While inspecting for muscle wasting in a patient who presents with a cervical spine complaint, the examiner must look not only at the wasting in and about the shoulder, but also distally in the hand. To ensure a comprehensive examination, the examiner should inspect for all features listed below on each side, as well as above and below the problem area.

Dividing the anatomy into regions—anterior, posterior, medial, and lateral ——facilitates a thorough, organized approach. Examining the shoulder only while standing behind the patient could be misleading, but beginning from this perspective is often helpful (**Fig. 3-12**). The examiner should move to the side, to the front, and, if possible, look down from above. Dividing the anatomy into soft tissue and bone further organizes the approach. In examining an anatomic region, a systematic inspection should routinely be performed for each of the following features, regardless of the part or complaint with different emphasis in different situations: attitude, alignment, color, swelling, deformities, muscle bulk and contour, and skin manifestations.

The patient with knee pain should be examined for attitude, alignment, deformities, and muscles in both the standing and the supine positions.

During inspection, the patient's position varies with the complaint and the presentation. Different features can be examined in different positions. For example, alignment of the lower extremities is examined in both the standing and supine positions.

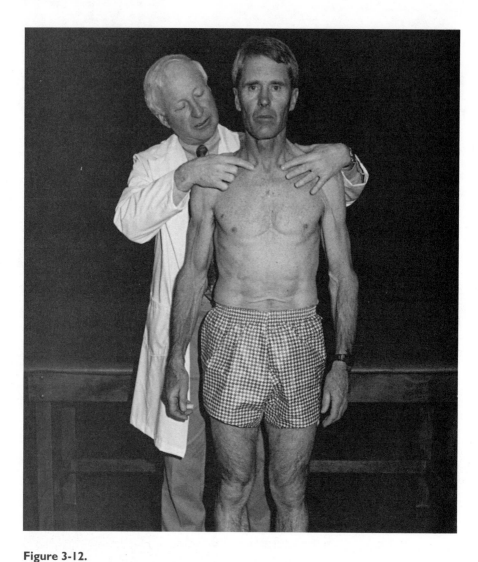

Figure 3-12.
The anatomy must be divided into regions such as anterior,
posterior, medial, and lateral. It is often helpful, for example,
in the shoulder girdle examination to commence the examination while standing behind the patient.

Attitude

This is the position in which the patient holds the
involved part relative to the body and the posture of the
segment in that position. It is demonstrated in the
slightly flexed posture of a septic knee (**Fig. 3-13**) or

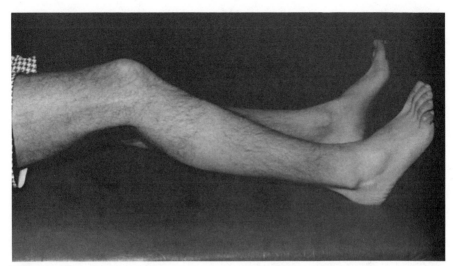

Figure 3-13.
The patient has a flexed attitude consistent with a septic knee.

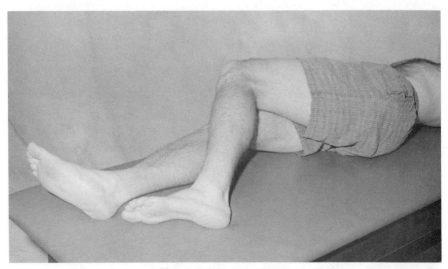

Figure 3-14.
The patient with a dislocated hip presents with the involved extremity shortened and internally rotated, lying across the opposite extremity. Ascribing malalignment to the hip is difficult, but malalignment can be ascribed to the extremity distal to the hip.

the internally rotated, adducted posture of a posterior dislocation of the hip **(Fig. 3-14)**, or the adducted, internally rotated position of a painful shoulder **(see Fig. 2-2)**. This position often provides a clue as to the degree of pain and disability and maybe the diagnosis. Attitude is influenced by pain, swelling, or an old malunited fracture producing a fixed deformity. Although frequently awkward, the examiner can duplicate a patient's attitude by positioning his extremities in the same position as the patient's. Listing of the spine due to low back pain or a torticollis deformity due to an atlantoaxial rotary fixation each present with a characteristic attitude. Examiners can duplicate the torticollis of atlantoaxial rotatory fixation with their own necks. This distinction is offered to emphasize that attitude differs from alignment.

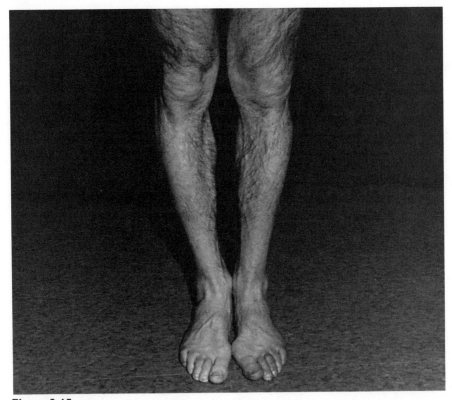

Figure 3-15.
The patient demonstrates a mild genu varum alignment of the knees and a significant hallux valgus alignment, particularly of the left foot.

Alignment

In extremities such as the arm and leg, or midline structures such as the spine, alignment varying from normal (i.e., malalignment) may be noted. Deformities such as genu varum **(Fig. 3-15)**, genu valgum, or cubitus valgus are relevant to the longitudinal segment of the extremity. Varus or valgus in the lower extremities can be documented by measuring the distance between the femoral condyles or malleoli **(Fig. 3-16)**. Terminology related to alignment can be confusing. A varus deformity is defined as one in which the distal segment is deviated toward the midline, whereas a valgus deformity is defined as one in which the distal segment is deviated away from the midline. In the lower extremity, this may be confusing because of what is considered the midline. Occasionally, the varus and valgus descriptions are inaccurate, but by convention are understood. For example, the term *genu varum* is accepted such that the segment distal to the knee is deviated toward the midline. Careful analysis of the phrase, however, shows that it is not the genu or knee that is deviated toward the midline; in fact, the knee is deviated away from the midline and perhaps would be more accurately termed genu valgum. In orthopedics, we are stuck with sometimes misleading descriptive terminology.

With central structures such as the shoulder or hip, ascribing malalignment is awkward, but more often one can refer to malalignment distal to these structures. For example, a dislocated hip is described as lying in the malaligned position of internal rotation and shortening **(Fig. 3-14)**. This probably more accurately represents attitude rather than malalignment. Unlike attitude, if the patient has malalignment of a part, a normal individual would have difficulty duplicating that position, although with difficulty, individuals with straight legs can position their knees into a genu varum position. This represents an exaggerated situation.

Different positions of an extremity may change alignment. For example, a gun stock deformity may not be obvious until the patient straightens his arm. Similarly, a patient with significant lateral knee instability may have a much more accentuated varus deformity on standing, compared with the supine position. While walking, this deformity may be further accentuated in

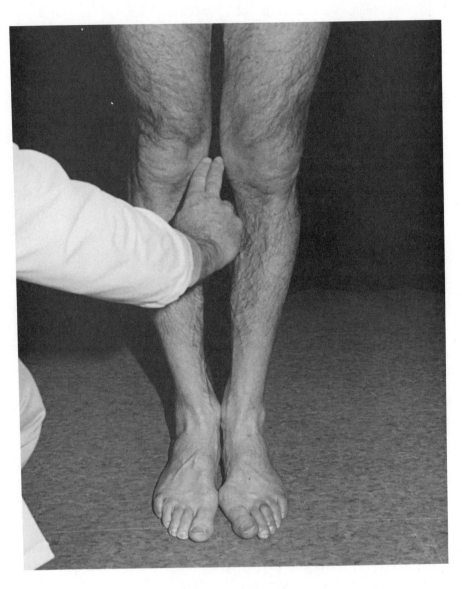

Figure 3-16.
Varus or valgus of the knees is documented by measuring the distance between the femoral condyles or malleoli, respectively. The patient has a varus alignment allowing two fingers between the femoral condyles.

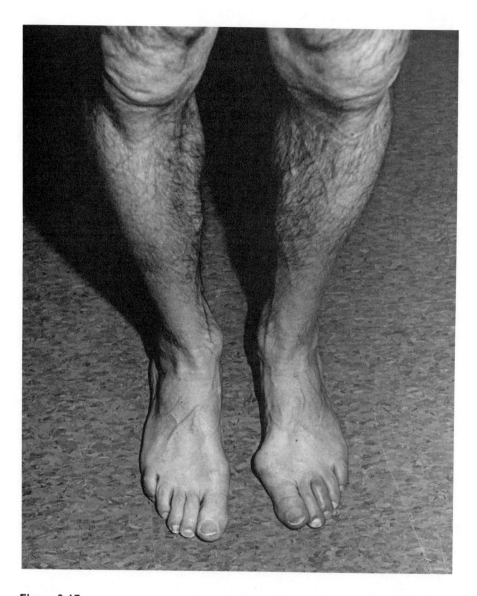

Figure 3-17.
Alignment terms in the foot can be confusing, depending on what is accepted as the midline. The patient demonstrates a significant hallux valgus alignment of the great toe of the left foot.

the form of a lateral thrust, which is an increase in the varus malalignment. Alignment terms in the foot can be confusing, depending upon what is accepted as the midline—the second toe or between the feet (Fig. 3-17). If the second toe is accepted as the midline, as in Fig. 3-17, hallux valgus is somewhat of a misnomer because the distal part is not in valgus, but rather in varus. By convention, however, this has been accepted as a hallux valgus deformity. Perhaps the bunion itself is in valgus, whereas the distal part is in varus. We consider not only alignment of straight structures such as upper and lower extremities, but also midline structures such as the spine, which might reveal a scoliosis or accentuated lumbar lordosis, each representing malalignment.

Color

Bruising is indicative of underlying bleeding suggesting a disruption of soft tissue or bone, such as in the upper arm following an injury to the shoulder from a rotator cuff tear or fracture. An ankle sprain frequently evolves through a rainbow of colors from initial redness to purple, often with hints of yellow and green. The observation of ecchymosis in the popliteal fossa in a patient who has sustained a dislocated knee suggests an underlying arterial disruption, which is critical to appreciate. So, too, is the determination of pulses distal to a vascular injury (Fig. 3-18).

Swelling

While swelling is noted visually, further characterization and quantification must await palpation. For example, synovial hypertrophy may visually masquerade as a joint effusion and remain undetermined until palpated.

Swelling that occurs at a joint is particularly common in the knee and ankle, but not so obvious in joints such as the hip or shoulder. Nevertheless, physicians do see swelling such as a fluid sign in the shoulder in patients with rheumatoid arthritis and bursal swelling (Fig. 3-19). Occasionally, a peculiar, enlarged cystic swelling may appear over the shoulder from a ruptured rotator cuff and leakage of the fluid into the subacromial bursa. Swelling may occur in concert with an infection from a joint or in the midshaft of the tibia from

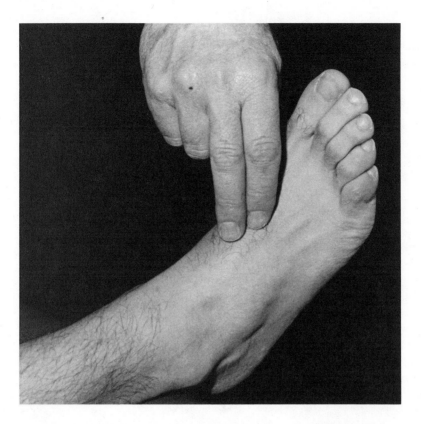

Figure 3-18.
Determination of peripheral pulses distal to the level of an extremity lesion is critical but is not the only assessment of vascularity.

an osteomyelitis. Swelling can extend above and below from the point of pathology. Similarly, a hematoma in the thigh from a femoral fracture can grossly enlarge the thigh. The combined visual inspection signs of marked swelling and significant redness in a joint may strongly suggest an underlying infection, or at least a significant inflammatory reaction.

The swelling that onsets immediately following a twisting injury to a knee presenting with a tense hemarthrosis is often due to an anterior cruciate ligament tear **(Fig. 3-20)**. Special tests can be performed to assess the amount of fluid in the knee. **Figs.** 3-21, A, B demonstrate a milking maneuver by initially

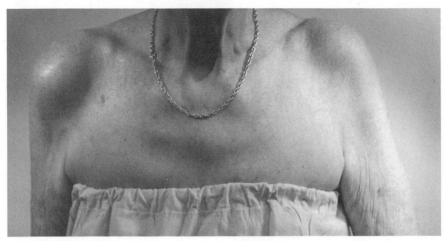

Figure 3-19.
Although swelling is uncommon in the shoulder, this patient
with rheumatoid arthritis demonstrates bursal swelling.

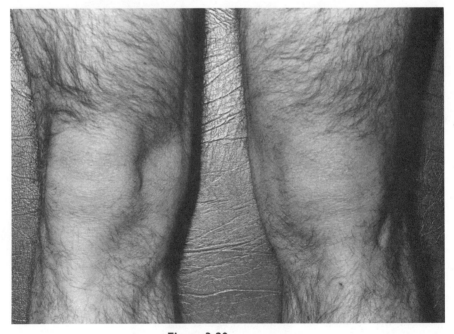

Figure 3-20.
Knee swelling following an acute injury is often suggestive of
an anterior cruciate ligament tear.

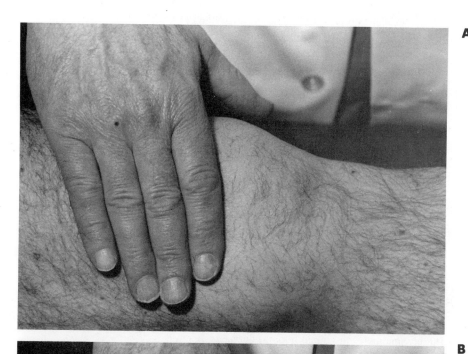

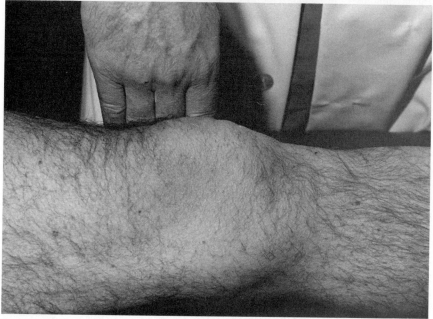

Figure 3-21.

A, B, Special tests described with the knee demonstrate various amounts of fluid.

forcing the fluid up into the suprapatellar pouch and then by bringing the hand down, the lateral aspect of the knee, looking for a fluid bulge medially. This represents 20 to 30 ccs of fluid in a knee joint. **Fig.** 3-22 demonstrates ballottement of the patella, suggesting 40 to 50 ccs of fluid.

Deformities

Some aspects of physical examination are difficult to categorize and can be combined under the term *deformities.* These include obvious anomalies such as absent parts (e.g., an amputated limb) or large tumors. They also include more subtle superficial abnormalities such as lacerations, scars, lumps, or cysts **(Figs. 3-23, 3-24).** A disturbance of architecture such as a high-riding scapula as in Sprengel's deformity or a mishapened knee with a dislocated patella might be described under deformities.

Scars, when present from previous operations or injuries, are significant deformities **(Figs. 3-25, 3-26).** The presence of scars about a joint may be associated with a history related to previous surgical intervention

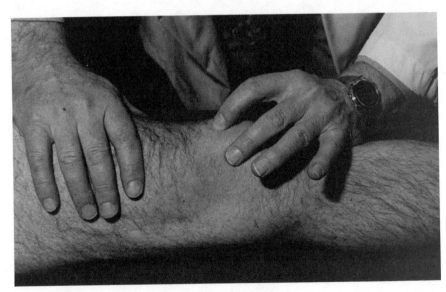

Figure 3-22.
Pateller ballottement demonstrates approximately 40 to 50 ccs of fluid.

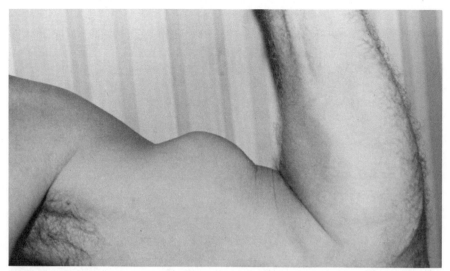

Figure 3-23.
The examiner should inspect for deformities. If a ruptured
biceps muscle is suspected, the patient is asked to contract
his biceps, thereby illustrating the popeye deformity.

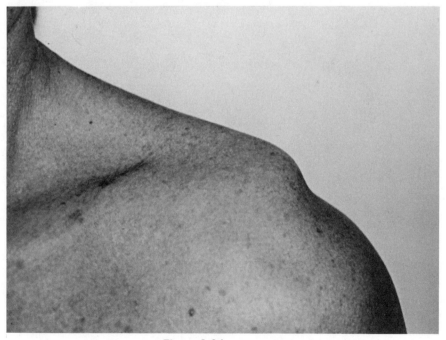

Figure 3-24.
A patient with an old acromioclavicular dislocation presents
with a high-riding clavicle, an obvious deformity.

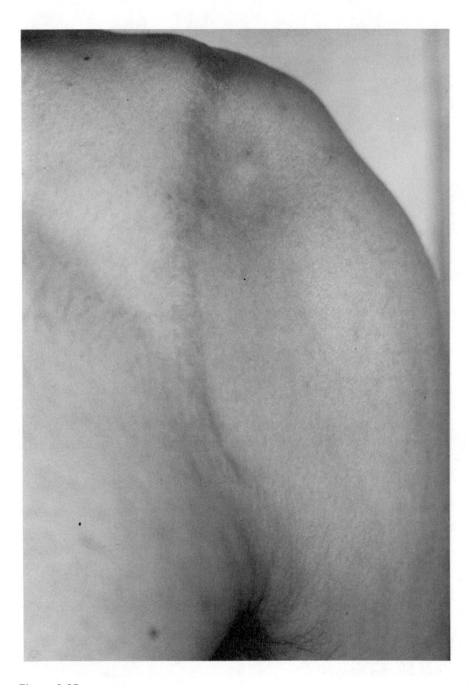

Figure 3-25.
A deformity such as a scar over the anterior aspect of the
shoulder is a telltale sign of previous surgery.

or injury. Scars may provide clues relating to the patient's tissue, such as whether they are keloid formers or have some form of collagen deficiency manifest with spreading of a scar. Other skin abnormalities may be present as well, such as abnormal hair distribution or patches. The entire extremity may be deformed following a brachial plexus lesion such as with Erb's or Klumpke's palsies. Winging of the scapula is an interesting deformity, often evident only with certain testing positions such as pushing the outstretched arms against a wall (**Fig. 3-27**). Therefore, certain visual deformities may only be evident with change of position or with provocative testing.

Through inspection plus palpation, each deformity must be carefully considered for characteristics of shape, location, consistency, and tenderness. The physician should attempt to quantitate certain deformities, such as determining the size of a nodule.

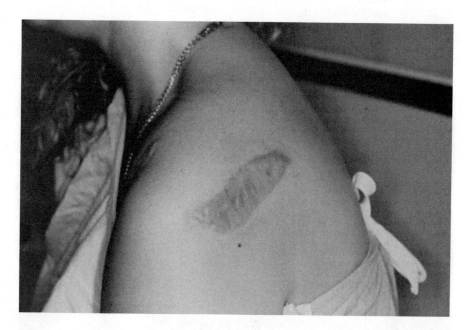

Figure 3-26.
This young female patient demonstrates a very spread scar following posterior reconstruction for her shoulder instability. The scar raises concerns about some form of collagen abnormality, which might suggest the reason the reconstruction failed.

Muscle Bulk and Contour

Muscle variation in the form of wasting is a frequent accompaniment of many disease processes. Muscle wasting may be noted localized to the part such as thigh atrophy with a meniscal tear in the knee, or it may be more generalized in the extremity such as entire lower extremity wasting as in osteoarthritis of the hip. In a patient with neck and arm pain, enlargement of the paracervical muscles due to spasm and pain may be observed; at the same time interosseous wasting distally in the hand due to a seventh cervical (C7) root lesion may also be observed. Muscular enlargement or prominence due to pain and spasm is particularly relevant to midline spinal pain. Because neurological compromise may affect muscle wasting, a careful neurological assessment is essential with its presence.

Muscle wasting can be a particularly helpful and often reliable physical sign suggesting a diagnosis. A 60-year-old patient presenting with shoulder pain who has localized infraspinatus wasting very probably has a rotator cuff defect **(Fig. 3-28)**. Deltoid wasting is a manifestation of axillary nerve deficiency **(Figs. 3-29,**

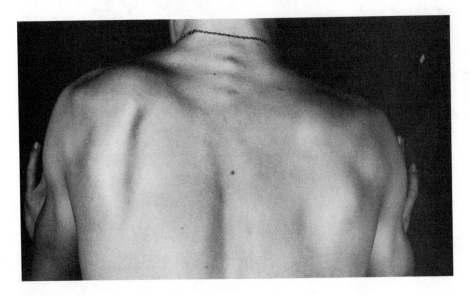

Figure 3-27.
Deformities such as scapular winging often can be illustrated only with provocative maneuvers. The patient is demonstrating left scapular winging by pushing the arms forward against the wall.

A, B). Similarly, patients who have a long-standing meniscal tear almost always have wasting of the thigh with loss of quadriceps bulk and contour. Marked interosseous wasting of the hand suggests either a C7 root lesion of the cervical spine or a peripheral ulnar lesion. Patients with osteoarthritis of the hip present with diffuse buttock and thigh wasting. Even an L5 root lesion in the back, if long-standing, can present distally in the foot with loss of bulk of the extensor brevis muscle.

To assess muscle bulk, having the patient contract a muscle or group of muscles is helpful. Contraction also allows the examiner to observe tone and contour while indirectly providing an assessment of strength. Importantly, certain deformities such as a quadriceps tear or biceps rupture become evident only on contraction of the quadriceps or biceps (Fig. 3-23).

Therefore, when examining the knee in an athletic individual, the examiner may find that asking the patient to contract his quads by pushing his knees into the bed, thereby allowing comparison of each side, helpful. By doing this, the examiner looks for bulk and contour, particularly of the vastus medialis or any defects that may represent a tear of the quadriceps.

Skin Manifestations

A general evaluation of skin condition completes our visual inspection of the part. Diabetic ulceration and fragility of the skin in the rheumatoid population have both local and systemic implications. Skin manifestations may suggest a vascular abnormality, which has a separate section in this format.

Patients may present with a patch of hair or a nevus discoloration. Shiny skin or sweating may suggest reflex dystrophy. A café au lait spot is interesting pathology that may come under deformities, but it also might be described under skin manifestations.

Inspecting the joints above and below the area of complaint for any abnormalities is appropriate at this stage. Sometimes abnormalities occur far removed from this area. For example, while directing attention toward the chief complaint of knee pain, a midline scar in the chest from open-heart surgery or obvious rheumatoid deformities in the hand may be observed (Fig. 3-30). By inspecting the joints above and below the

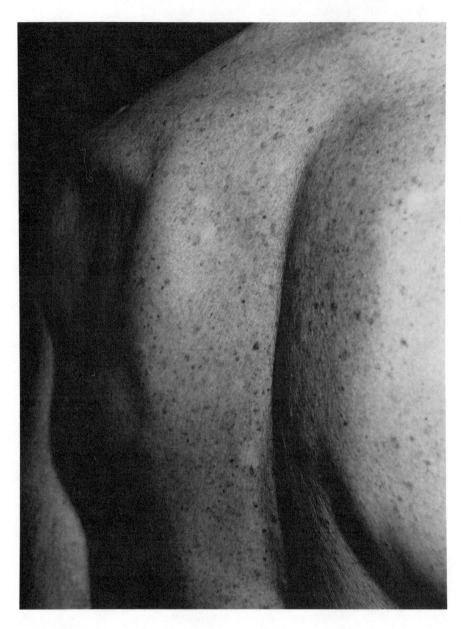

Figure 3-28.
Muscle wasting is a tell-tale sign of either a musculotendinous rupture or a neurologic deficiency. This 60-year-old
patient demonstrates significant infraspinatus wasting that,
with the appropriate findings, is strongly suggestive of a
complete thickness rotator cuff tear.

area of complaint as well as the joints farther afield, that part of the examination can be completed at this time, thereby avoiding subsequently doubling back.

The duration of time required for inspection depends on the experience and thoroughness of the examiner, the pathology that may be present, and, to some degree, the patient. With experience, however, the pathological findings on inspection can be rapidly assimilated.

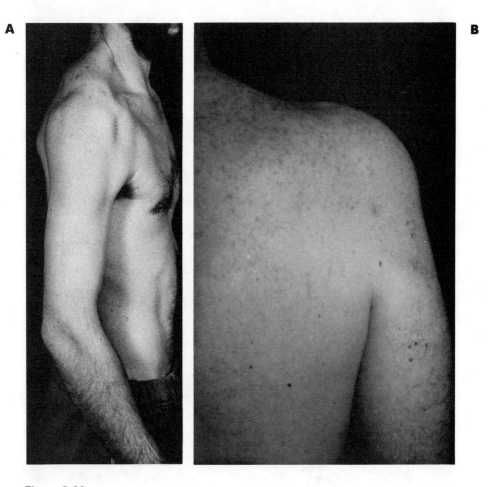

Figure 3-29.
A, Deltoid wasting visualized either from the front, the side, or the back, is often a manifestation of an axillary nerve deficiency. B, Other causes for such deltoid wasting, such as a brachial plexus injury or a cervical spine problem, must also be considered.

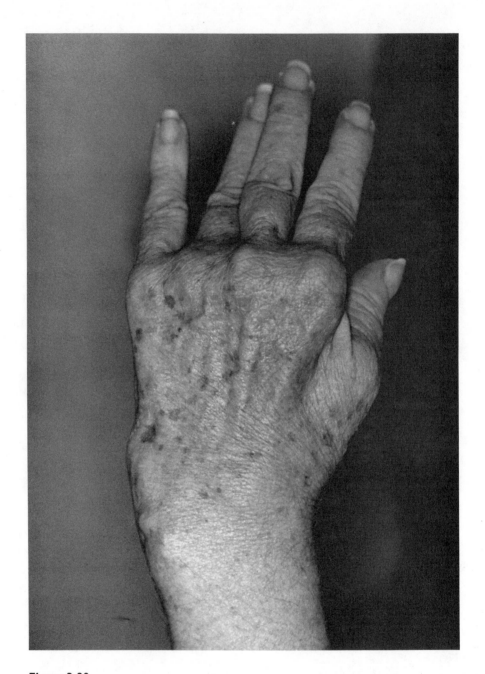

Figure 3-30.
By directing attention toward the chief complaint of knee pain, the examiner might observe obvious rheumatoid deformities in the hand, which might suggest an etiology for the knee pain.

Palpation

Palpation prior to visual inspection is inappropriate because it may focus the examiner's attention too narrowly. Most of that which was visually inspected should now be palpated. As with inspection, the part to be examined should be divided into regions such as anterior, posterior, medial, and lateral. Further division into bone and soft tissue architecture within each region is helpful.

During palpation, many features are noted simultaneously. Palpation truly represents the art of the examination and during palpation one often appreciates the phrase describing the examiner as having "sensitive fingers." Examiners not only feel simultaneously for many features such as temperature, swelling, and deformity, but they also note that the structures are all present and the architecture is in its appropriate relationship. This is frequently done very quickly by simply placing the examiner's hand on a part. Examiners also need to apply pressure to different areas, particularly in eliciting tenderness and looking for hidden deformities in the depths of muscular tissue. Although many aspects of palpation are done simultaneously, they will be considered individually as follows: architecture, temperature, swelling, muscle features, deformity, and tenderness.

Architecture

In examining a patient who has had previous knee surgery, the examiner may not find evidence that a patellectomy was performed without palpating for its absence. Also, only on palpation might the examiner find evidence that a tumor is hidden deep in muscle.

Temperature

Temperature is frequently determined by the examiner placing the backs of the hands on the affected part and comparing the two sides. Temperature is vitally important; a warm or hot knee on one side might suggest referral to a rheumatologist rather than an orthopedic surgeon. Infections and inflammatory reactions frequently accompany increased temperature. Hemoarthrosis and patients in the immediate postoperative period in different parts and joints of the body frequently have increased temperature to that part.

Swelling

Although swelling may have been observed on inspection, determining its features and cause without palpation is difficult **(Figs. 3-19, 3-20)**. The swelling may be soft tissue swelling as in cellulitis, it may be bony as in generalized osteophyte formation, or it may be caused by fluid. The type of fluid within the joint (e.g., synovial fluid, blood, or pus) each has its own characteristics. Specific tests applied to the knee can determine the amount of synovial fluid that may be present. An example of such a test is the milking technique that consists of pushing the fluid into the suprapatellar pouch and demonstrating a fluid bulge by pushing it back into the main knee joint from the opposite side, which demonstrates approximately 15 to 20 ccs of fluid within the knee **(Figs. 3-21, A, B)**. Other methods to estimate the amount of fluid are tests such as patellar ballottement **(Fig. 3-22)**, patellar tap, or simply the feeling or fluctuance with fingers on each side of the joint.

The consistency of the fluid should be noted. Pus has a thick consistency and is less fluctuant than synovial fluid. Hematoma may become gel-like in consistency. Swelling is much more pertinent to certain areas such as the knee and ankle. Swelling that follows an acute ankle sprain is different than that following an anterior cruciate ligament tear in the knee. The swelling following an ankle sprain is rather diffuse and nonfluctuant soft tissue, whereas the knee ligament sprain is much more fluctuant. Tenderness may be associated with swelling due to distention of a part such as the capsule of a joint.

Muscle Features

Changes in muscles can be localized and generalized and can affect individual muscles or groups of muscles. Changes may be related to a joint or occur between joints. Palpating both the relaxed and the contracted muscles allows an appreciation of bulk and tone and also allows assessment of any deformity such as a rupture **(Fig. 3-23)** or tumor that may be present. Muscle wasting is often very meaningful; for example, infraspinatus wasting in an older individual with shoulder pain is strongly suggestive of a rotator cuff tear **(Fig. 3-28)**. Spastic enlarged or prominent muscles are very hard and frequently tender to palpation. Trigger areas along various muscles are common, especially along trapezius and rhomboids. The examiner often makes an assessment that if a patient can bulk up his muscle affectively equal to the opposite side, then it carries some connotation suggesting normal strength. In palpating the muscles, the examiner not only feels for bulk and tone, but also for tenderness and defects. Fibrillation fasciculation or tremors related to muscles might indicate neurologic disease. The examiner must palpate deep into muscle areas to be as certain as possible that no underlying deformity exists such as a tumor.

Deformities

Any deformities that were visually inspected in addition to those present but not visually inspected should be palpated for their various characteristics. Defects such as scars **(Figs. 3-25, 3-26)**, lacerations, lumps, or bumps **(Figs. 3-23, 3-24)** should be analyzed with regard to location, size, and characteristics such as tenderness or fluctuance. Generalized deformities may occur as in the rheumatoid hand **(Fig. 3-30)**. Scapular winging may represent a deformity **(Figs. 3-31, 3-32)**. A hidden deformity such as an osteochondroma or a soft tissue tumor may only be realized by deep palpation of the area. In palpating a tumor, the examiner should carefully consider its size, location, consistency, and tenderness (if any). If a patient has a scar, the examiner may palpate along the scar for its consistency, particularly looking for any areas of tenderness that might indicate an underlying neuroma.

Tenderness

Assessment of tenderness is critically important and may be one of the most important physical signs

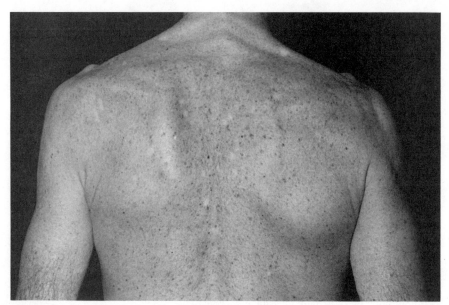

Figure 3-31.
Scapular winging may represent a deformity and can often be
very subtle, as illustrated.

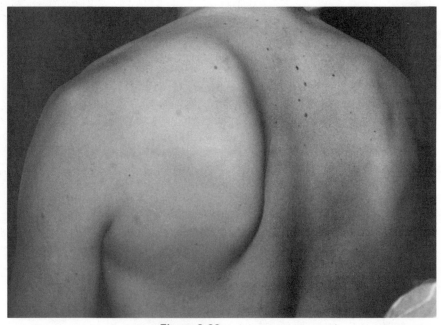

Figure 3-32.
Scapular winging can also be very dramatic in the resting
state, as shown with significant winging of the left scapula.

relating to pathology **(Figs. 3-33 to 3-35)**. Knowing the anatomy and knowing what specific disease processes occur in those areas provides an appreciation of what specific areas to palpate. In palpating for tenderness, the examiner should not palpate generally; he must be specific in his actions. For example, a suspected meniscal tear in the knee should reveal joint line tenderness **(Fig. 3-36)**. Nevertheless, although the examiner knows the anatomic structures and potential common pathologies, he must still palpate generally for hidden pathologies such as tumors, trigger points of tenderness, or any other architectural abnormalities. Nowhere is having an organized systematic regional

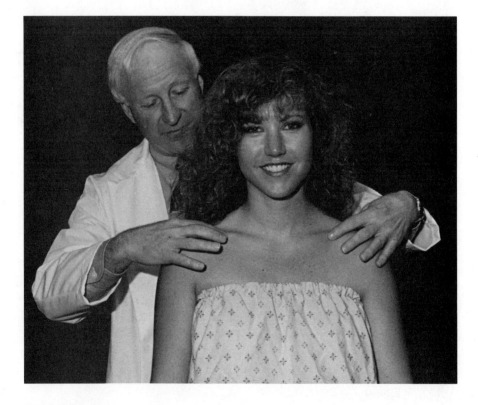

Figure 3-33.
Tenderness needs to be elicited at presentation, based on an organized approach to physical examination. Looking for any signs of tenderness, the examiner commences medially at the sternoclavicular joint and palpates along the clavicles of this young female patient.

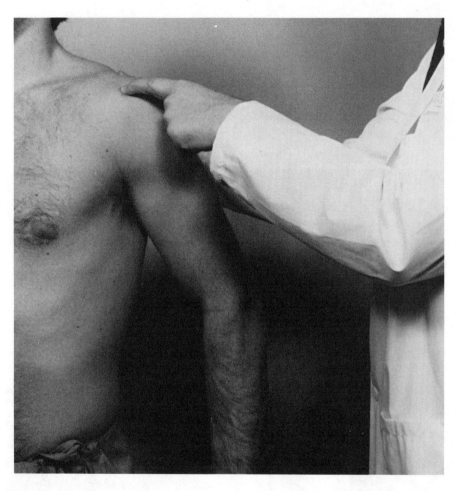

Figure 3-34.
By extending the upper arm slightly, the greater tuberosity is brought forward to the anterior acromion and is easily palpated for any tenderness.

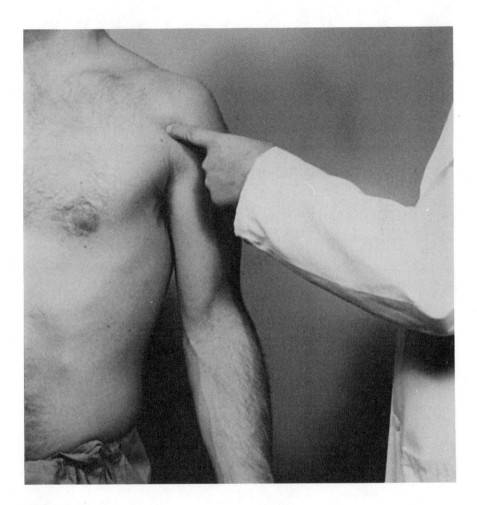

Figure 3-35.
By supinating the forearm, the area of the biceps tendon is palpated approximately 1 to 2 inches distal to the anterior acromion between the axillary fold and lateral border of the arm.

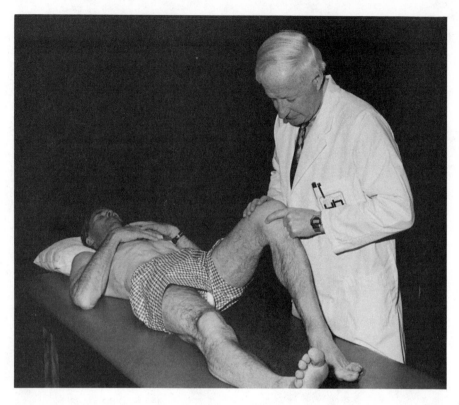

Figure 3-36.
A patient with a medial meniscal tear of the knee will almost always have medial joint line tenderness.

approach along with a division into bone and soft tissue more important **(Fig. 3-33)**. To ensure ongoing cooperation, especially with children, deferring palpation for tenderness until the end of the examination is often advisable.

Often the examiner may find that having the patient indicate where the pain is before beginning to palpate is helpful. For example, patients who suggest that they have shoulder pain may indicate pain coming from the trapezial area by placing a hand over this area **(Fig. 3-37, A)**. This probably indicates pain from a neck

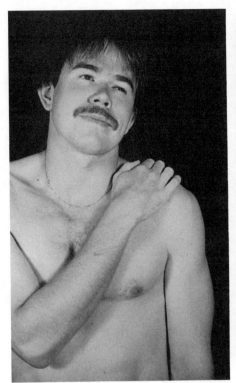
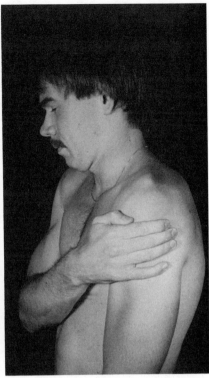

Figure 3-37.
A, Patients who have pain in the shoulder girdle that eminates from the cervical spine often place the hand over the top of the shoulder and trapezius. B, Those who have pain from the shoulder itself, such as rotator cuff tendinitis, often place the hand over the lateral aspect of the deltoid, indicating the site of pain.

problem. Similarly, a hand placed over the lateral deltoid may indicate a shoulder problem (**Fig. 3-37, B**).

The examiner must palpate for pulses distal to the area of concern. However, because of the importance and variations in the presentation of vascular problems, a separate chapter entitled Vascularity is included (see Chapter 9).

Chapter

4

Range of Motion

Having completed inspection and palpation, the physician now deviates from the classical method of physical examination by modifying the musculoskeletal system exam by next examining range of motion. The broad classification of range of motion is divided into active motion and passive motion. *Active motion* is the range produced by the patient (**Fig. 4-1**). *Passive motion* is the range produced by the examiner (**Figs. 4-2, 4-3**). Specific joints may vary as to the planes of motion and the ranges within each plane. The knee, for example, primarily goes through a range of flexion and extension from 0 degrees (straight) and flexes up to approximately 140 degrees limited by the buttock. The shoulder, conversely, is multiplanar in motion and which motions should be documented can be confusing. The physician should carefully describe the motion with which he is concerned. Terminology describing these planes of motion should be the same, even though different joints are being described. For example, rather than stating that the ankle goes into adduction when the forefoot deviates toward the midline, for consistency, the examiner should describe the motion as *internal rotation,* which is the term applied to other joints in the body (**Fig. 4-4**).

Where feasible, each motion should be documented by comparing contralateral sides or joints. With regard to the shoulder, stating that the shoulder externally rotates from 0 to 10 degrees without stating that the opposite side rotates from 0 to 70 degrees is inappropriate (**Fig. 4-5**). Comparison may only be important if the range of motion is not normal. The physician should consider the part, the motion, and the range of variation that may occur among individuals for that motion. For example, if a patient has full elevation, documenting the opposite side is not as critical, but still it should be considered. In bilateral disease, what is normal for that particular patient's joint, age, or disease might provide

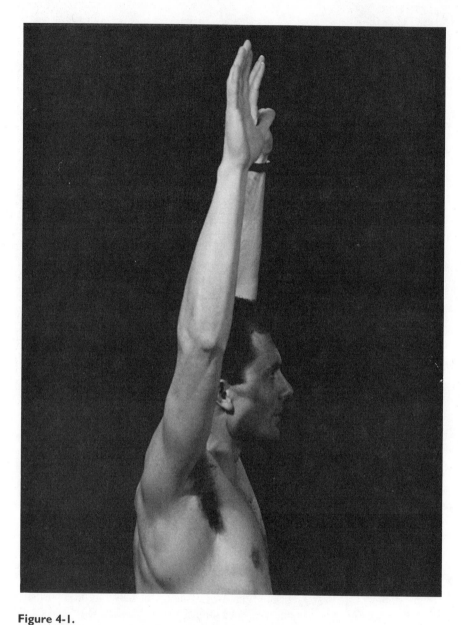

Figure 4-1.
Active range of motion is produced by the patient. When testing active motion, the patient's own muscle power completes the range of motion, here demonstrating forward elevation of the shoulders.

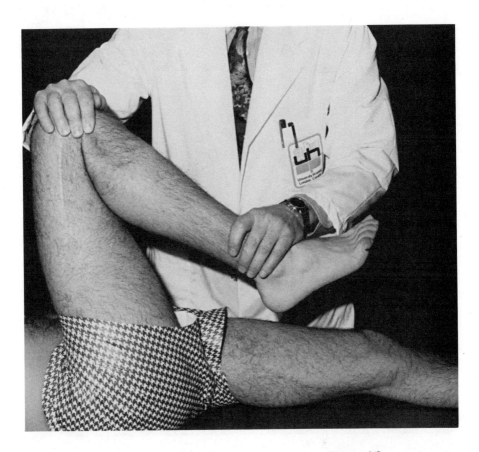

Figure 4-2.
Passive range of motion, here demonstrated for the knee and the hip, is produced by the examiner.

a benchmark for comparison. Sometimes, however, a comparison is impossible; for example, with extension of the lumbar spine, no bilateral application exists.

When testing active motion, the patient's own muscle power is used to complete the range of motion (Fig. 4-1). Passive testing is always performed by the examiner at the extremes of motion and in the situation when the patient has difficulty fully performing the active portion of the examination (Figs. 4-2, 4-3). Different diagnoses suggests that the emphasis of the examination may be more focused on the active rather than passive assessment. For example, with instability problems about the shoulder, most motions are performed actively, whereas with degenerative problems about the hip, most motions are performed passively. If the patient is able to perform a complete range of

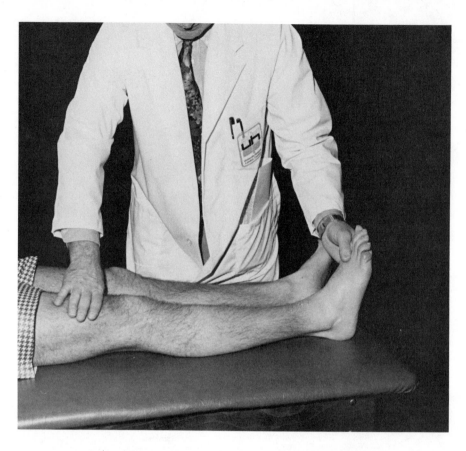

Figure 4-3.
Passive extension of the knee is demonstrated by the examiner, beginning at 0 degrees or full extension.

motion without pain, passive testing is not really needed, other than to stress the joint at the extremes of motion to elicit pain if it is present. When documenting any limitation of active or passive motion, the examiner should state whether the limitation is associated with pain, weakness, or deformity. Standard documentation is necessary for communication, follow-up, and research. Because functionally assessing certain motions is important, some parts require examination with the patient upright (such as range of motion of the lumbar spine), some sitting (such as range of motion of the shoulder), and others supine (such as range of motion of the hip) **(Fig. 4-6)**. Sometimes physicians may vary positions to analyze active motion in one position and passive motion in another position, such

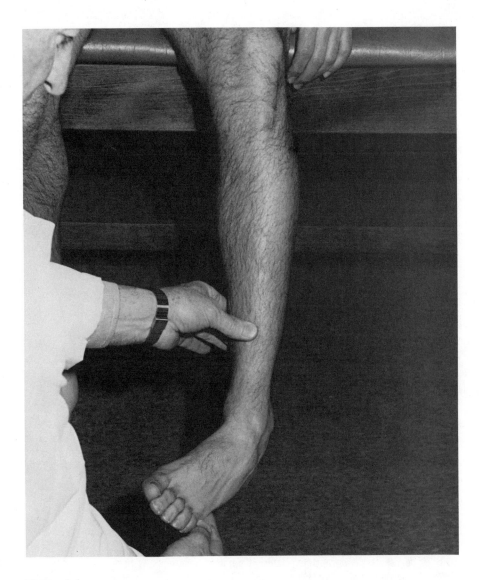

Figure 4-4.
Range of motion of the ankle can be confusing, but to ensure consistency with examination of the rest of the body, this motion should be described as internal rotation of the ankle, demonstrated passively.

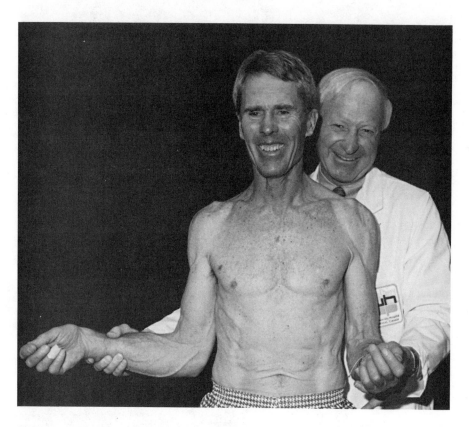

Figure 4-5.
This doctor is demonstrating external rotation. Documenting
external rotation of the left shoulder passively from 0 to 10
degrees without documenting the opposite normal side from
0 to 70 degrees is inappropriate. Different patients have
different degrees of normal external rotation.

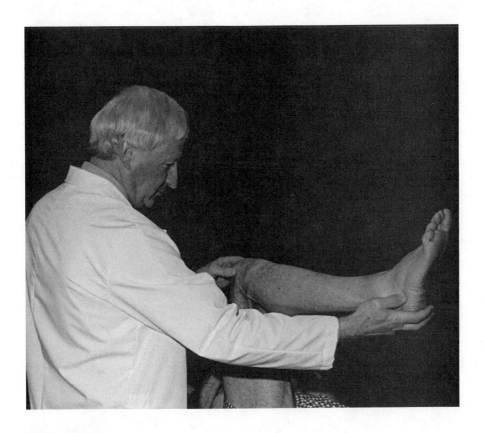

Figure 4-6.
Ranges of motion can be determined standing, sitting, or supine. Internal rotation of the hip is often determined supine.

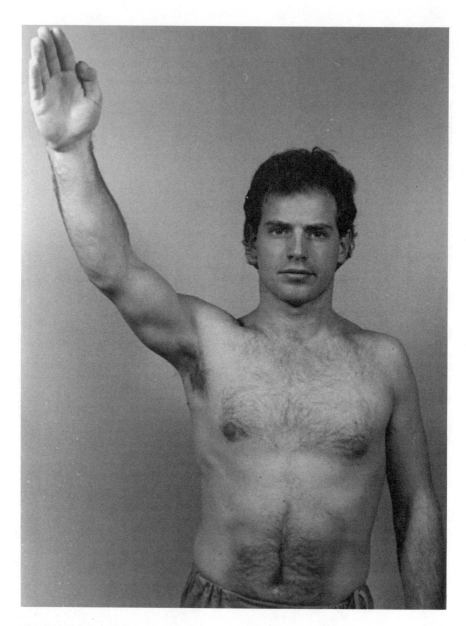

Figure 4-7.
Active elevation of the shoulder can be demonstrated standing or sitting.

as active elevation of the shoulder standing or sitting (Fig. 4-7) and passive elevation of the shoulder supine (Fig. 4-8). Eliminating compensatory movements above and below the part so as not to skew the results is important. For example, when observing shoulder elevation by asking the patient to elevate the arm in the frontal plane, the examiner must be careful to not allow any compensatory shifting of the thorax. To document abduction of the hip accurately, the physician needs to observe compensatory movements of the pelvis, identifying the plane of motion. With elevation of the shoulder, many planes are possible, such as forward in the sagittal plane and total elevation in the frontal plane (Fig. 4-9), the scapular plane, and the coronal plane (Fig. 4-10). Stating only the degree of elevation is not clear unless, by convention, the plane is already understood, but the examiner should carefully describe in what plane that elevation is occurring. Similarly, in describing external rotation of the shoulder, the exam-

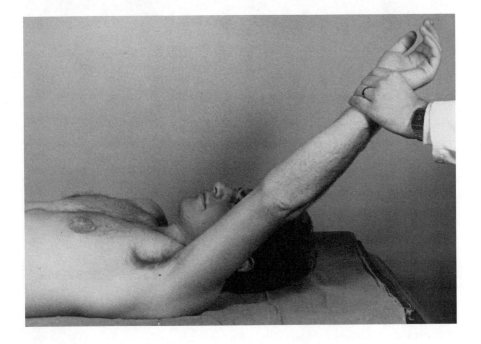

Figure 4-8.
Passive elevation of the shoulder may be determined supine.

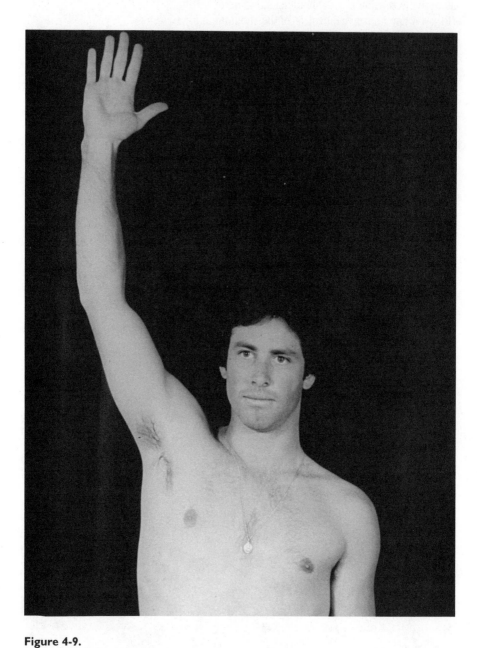

Figure 4-9.
This patient demonstrates total elevation in the frontal plane, which is midway between the sagittal and scapular planes. The frontal plane is the most comfortable for the patient to demonstrate and achieves the maximum amount of elevation.

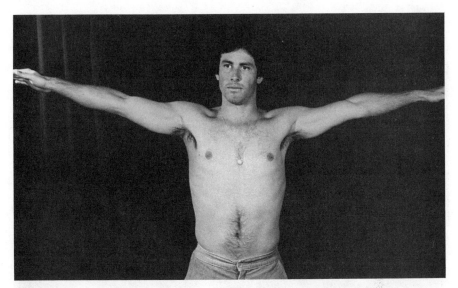

Figure 4-10.
Elevation in the coronal plane is not routinely documented but is routinely observed.

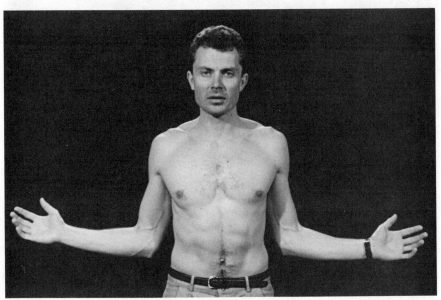

Figure 4-11.
This patient demonstrates active external rotation of the shoulder with arms at the sides and elbows slightly away from the body, revealing approximately 80 degrees of external rotation bilaterally.

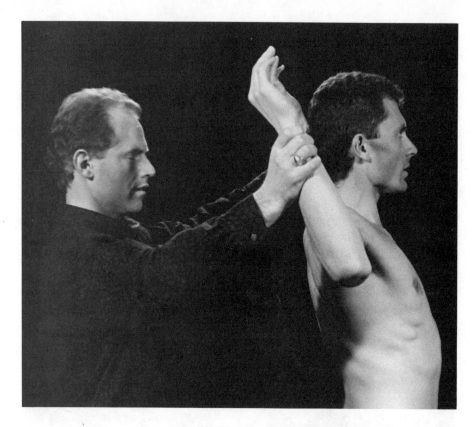

Figure 4-12.
External rotation is also documented in the 90-degree abducted position.

iner should be sure to note that it is with the arm at the side (Fig. 4-11) and, if not, define that it is in the 90 degree abducted position (Fig. 4-12).

Use of a Goniometer

For practical purposes most ranges are estimated by the examiner. However, certain circumstances and planes of motion should be measured with a goniometer. This is influenced by the part, the plane, the disease process, and perhaps the progression of the disease. In a patient with a postoperative flexion deformity of the knee, that deformity must be documented accurately (Fig. 4-13, A, B). In such a circumstance a goniometer is accurate, reliable, and reproducible. A goniometer is also useful when recording the angulation of a fracture with a fixed deformity. In these two circumstances, an accurate determination of angulation may direct treatment and allow serial mea-

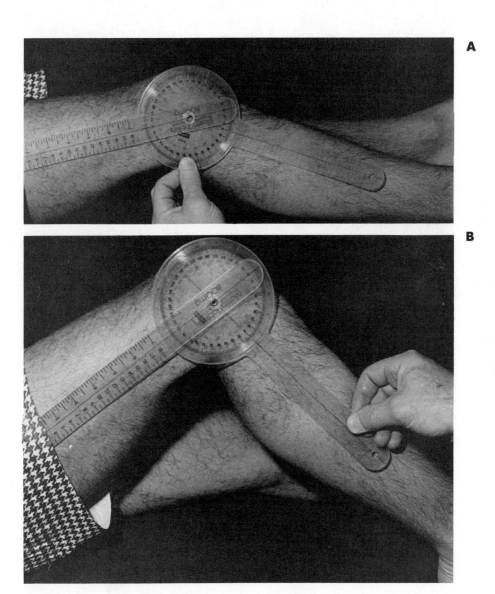

Figure 4-13.
A, B, In a patient with a postoperative flexion deformity of the knee, the physician must accurately document that deformity and how much flexion exists beyond the deformity. Using a goniometer is accurate, reliable, reproducible, and allows the physician to chart the disease process.

surements at different times to follow the progress of such a deformity. In analyzing external rotation of the shoulder with arms at the sides **(Fig. 4-11)** and in the 90 degree abducted position **(Fig. 4-12)**, planes relative to the floor and the body provide a reasonably accurate estimation of rotation. In such a circumstance, a goniometer is less necessary. Obviously, accurate scientific documentation of range would require a goniometer, but frequently it is not used in actual physical examination.

Active and passive motion of a joint may be documented by measurement by degrees, distances reached, and percentages of normal.

Measurement by Degrees

The accepted method for testing joint motion(s) is based on the principle of the neutral zero, first described by Cave and Roberts and approved in 1964 by the orthopedic associations of the English-speaking world. Simple, reliable, and reproducible, it permits comparisons to be made. Motion testing of various joints of each region of the body are described in subsequent chapters. In principle, the starting position is 0 degrees and not 180 degrees **(Figs. 4-3, 4-14)**. In a pathologic state and in some normal situations, the starting point may be other than zero degrees. This applies to both passive and active range of motion.

The general principles of measuring motion as defined by Cave and Roberts may be summarized as follows:

1. All motion should be measured by degrees from a neutral point of zero degrees.

2. The neutral points from which the motion is measured must be defined.

3. Comparative motions in the joint of the opposite limb should be mentioned.

4. When practical, angles should be measured with a goniometer or protractor.

5. Motions of joints above and below the affected part should be measured.

The specific motions of each region of the body are described in its respective section.

Measurement by degrees is the ideal and scientific method of measuring motion and should be appropriately recorded as such on the medical chart. For example, flexion of the knee may go through a range from 0 to 100 degrees actively and passively. In documenting degrees, straight is zero where applicable and when not applicable, the neutral position is the starting point of zero degrees (**Figs. 4-3, 4-14**). The starting point throughout the body differs from, but is very close to, the anatomical position. For example, the forearm and hands are examined with the forearm in neutral rotation, the palm against the lateral thigh, and the fingers extended. When documenting motion on the chart and for scientific purposes, each side must be

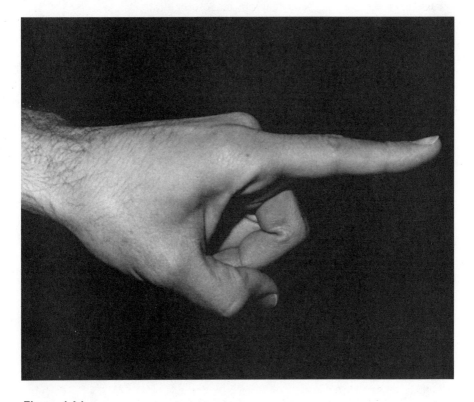

Figure 4-14.
This patient demonstrates the starting, or 0 degree, position for the metacarpo-phalangeal, proximal interphalangeal, and distal interphalangeal joints of the hand.

carefully documented from the starting point of neutral or zero. In verbal presentation, indicating how much motion the involved side lacks from the uninvolved side if the uninvolved side is normal may be easier.

In certain joints and motions, the physician must compare them to the opposite side. In scientific documentation, the physician begins at the zero or neutral point and measures from that point. In external rotation of the shoulder, for example, one might go from 0 to 10 degrees on one side and from 0 to 70 degrees on the opposite side (Fig. 4-5). Documenting only the pathological side could be misleading. In verbal presentation, for example, the physician might observe that the involved shoulder lacks 30 degrees of external rotation; inherent in such a statement is a comparison to the opposite normal shoulder.

Sometimes the starting point may not be zero or neutral, but a deformed position such as a 20 degree flexion deformity of the knee (Fig. 4-15). This position is not documented as 0 degrees but as 20 degrees and from there the physician documents whatever additional degrees are possible. This motion should be documented in degrees both actively and passively.

Sometimes the starting point of zero is very obvious, such as in the knee when it is straight. At other times, the zero degree starting point can be difficult to determine, such as a hip or shoulder, particularly in assessing rotation or abduction and adduction.

Sometimes ranges are documented in different positions. For example, hip rotation may be documented at 0 degrees and 90 degrees of flexion. External rotation of the shoulder is documented both in neutral, with the arm at the side (Fig. 4-11), and in the 90 degree abducted position (Fig. 4-12). Much variation is seen in the amount of external rotation in these two positions. A shoulder that has 45 degrees of external rotation at the side usually has 90 degrees of external rotation with the arm in the 90 degree abducted position. These are obviously measuring different aspects of rotation, and it relates to both normal and pathological situations.

Distances Reached

Certain assessments of joint motion do not permit evaluation in degrees because of the complex pattern and adjacent joint involvement. In such circumstances, using the reference of distance reached relative to an anatomical landmark may provide the best method of documentation. This approach may be applied to internal rotation of the shoulder, which is documented by the level of the spinous processes reached with the hitch-hiking thumb **(Fig. 4-16)**, or to flexion of the lumbar spine, which is assessed by the distance reached by the patient's fingertips relative to the toes **(Fig. 4-17)**. The floor could also be used as a reference, assuming it is flat. Cervical spine flexion can be documented relative to the number of fingerbreadths from the sternum that the chin can reach **(Fig. 4-18)**. Obviously, someone with a thick sternum or double chin may provide an erroneous measure. If possible and where applicable, the physician should document the contralateral side in an identical fashion.

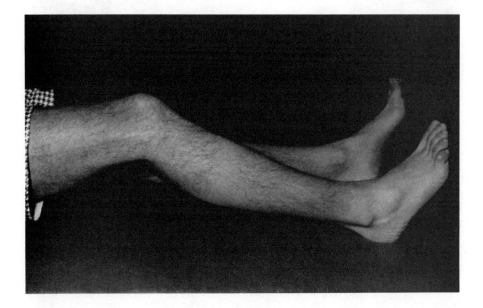

Figure 4-15.
Sometimes the starting point at which to examine a part is not zero, as in this knee, which has a flexion deformity of 20 degrees. Twenty degrees, then, represents the starting point to document flexion of the knee.

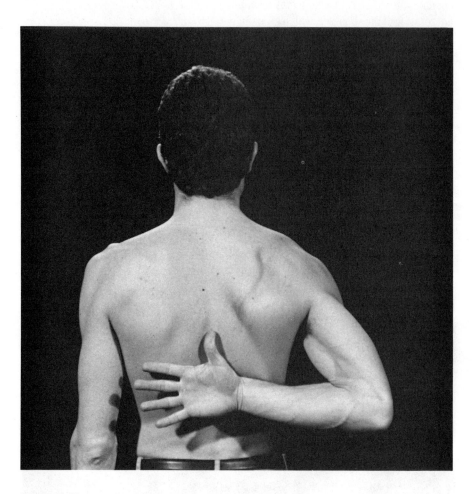

Figure 4-16.
Sometimes motion is documented by where a part reaches in reference to the patient's anatomy. Internal rotation of the shoulder is documented by noting where the tip of the hitchhiking thumb reaches relative to the spinous processes, such as here to T9.

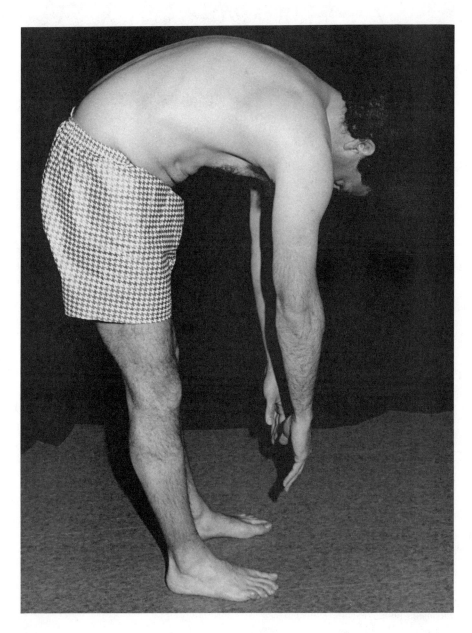

Figure 4-17.
Flexion of the lumbar spine may be assessed by where the
fingertips reach relative to one's anatomy or the distance
from the floor.

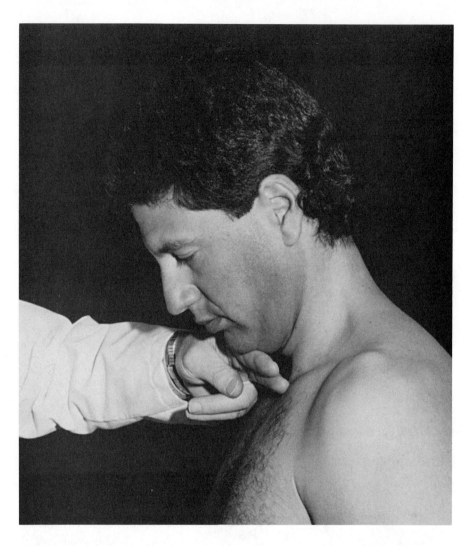

Figure 4-18.
Flexion of the chin can be
documented by the number
of fingerbreadths of chin to
sternum.

Percentages of Normal

This is the most subjective approach to measurement
of joint motion and should be reserved for axial movements that do not permit more accurate assessment.
For example, cervical spine extension is difficult to
assess except for comparison with normal, for example, 50% of normal **(Fig. 4-19)**. More refined
methods to document cervical spine extension exist,
such as considering the occipito-mental line, but this is
more applicable to scientific endeavors and probably
too complex for everyday clinical application. Lumbar

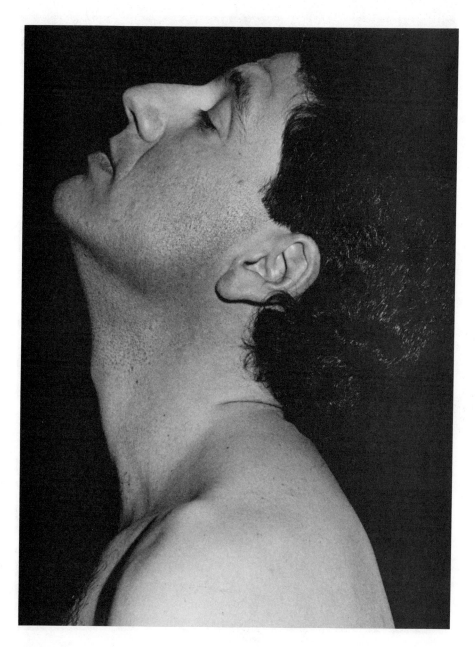

Figure 4-19.
Documenting some motions such as extension of the cervical spine is sometimes difficult. This patient has a 50% limitation of cervical spine extension.

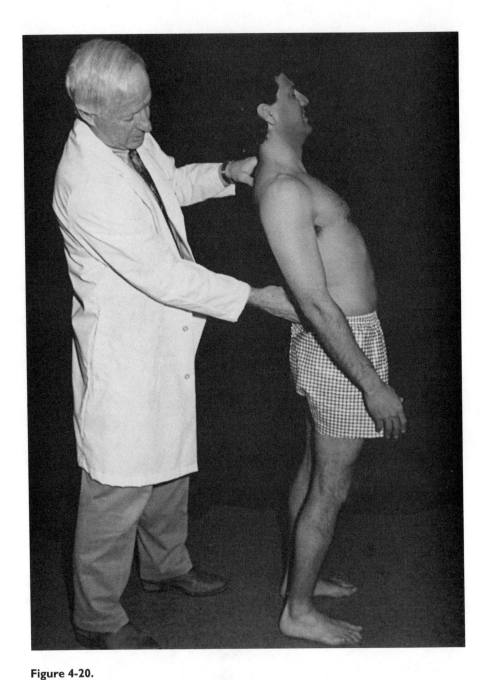

Figure 4-20.

In the lumbar spine, accurately documenting what is considered normal, unrestricted extension is difficult; however, in this patient, it is moderately restricted and painful.

and thoracic spine extension likewise are motions where some estimate of the percentage of normal might be applied or some other method of estimation might be suggested, such as whether extension is mildly or moderately restricted (Fig. 4-20). Unfortunately, this method suffers from subjectivity and varies among examiners, but is probably the best available. The examiner should remember that describing a patient as having mildly restricted motion may in fact be normal for that particular patient.

Planes of Motion

Different joints go through different motions; for example, the knee moves only through flexion and extension, whereas the shoulder, being multiplanar, moves in many directions. Measuring and documenting all of these motions in some joints would be impossible. By convention and agreement, most have standardized motions that are measured (e.g., hip, knee, ankle).

Table 4-1 describes orthopedic definitions for positions and deviations, most of which represent motions. Others represent a definition of a position; for example, kyphosis. Some can be defined as both a motion and as a position, for example, the motion of supination of the forearm versus the position of supination of the forefoot in a clubfoot deformity. These terms are applied interchangeably and often inaccurately, which sometimes leads to confusion.

Motions Considered at Each Joint

Standardized motions must be documented for each joint. This allows a method of communication, provides objectivity, and provides a means of producing outcome studies.

Cervical Spine

By convention, the motions to be documented in the cervical spine are flexion (Fig. 4-18), extension (Fig. 4-19), lateral flexion (Fig. 4-21), and rotation (Fig. 4-22). Cervical spine flexion is documented by the number of fingers from the sternum reached by the chin, extension by an estimate of some nature, lateral flexion by degrees from the midline, and rotation by degrees from the midline. A goniometer is not practical for cervical spine motion.

TABLE 4-1
STANDARD ORTHOPEDIC DEFINITIONS
FOR POSITIONS AND DEVIATIONS

Terms	Definition
Abduction	To draw away or deviate from the midline of the body
Adduction	To deviate or draw toward the midline of the body
Eversion	Turning outward
Extension	The act of straightening; when the part distal to a joint extends it straightens
External rotation	Rotatory motion in the transverse plane away from the midline
Flexion	The act or condition of being bent; when a joint is flexed the part distal to the joint bends
Internal rotation	Rotatory motion in the transverse plane toward the midline
Inversion	Turning inward
Kyphosis	An increased rounding of the normal thoracic curve of the spine
Lordosis	The anterior concavity in the curvature of the lumbar and cervical spines when viewed from the side
Pronation	Assuming a prone position is applied to the foot, it refers to a combination of eversion and abduction movements resulting in a lowering of the medial margin of the foot; applied to the forearm, it assumes a turning downward of the palm of the hand
Supination	The act of assuming a supine position; applied to the foot, it refers to a raising of the medial margin of the foot; applied to the palm of the hand, it refers to a turning of the palm upward
Varus*	Refers to deviation of a portion of an extremity distal to a joint away from the midline of the body
Valgus*	Refers to deviation of a portion of the extremity distal to a joint toward the midline of the body

*Valgus and varus are often used in the vernacular to describe the deformity of a fracture site wherein the part distal to a fracture is away or toward the midline of the body, respectively.

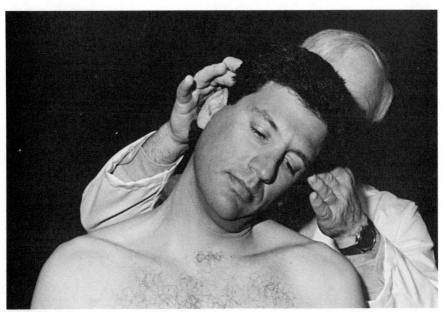

Figure 4-21.
Lateral flexion is determined in the cervical spine by degrees
from the midline.

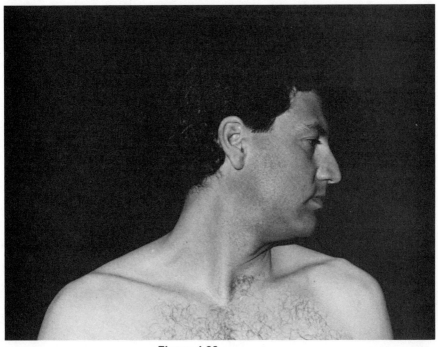

Figure 4-22.
Rotation is determined in the cervical spine by degrees from
the midline.

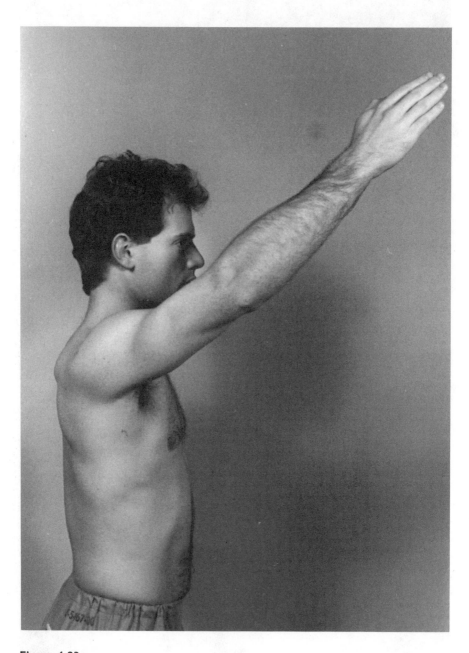

Figure 4-23.
Active forward elevation in the frontal plane of 145 degrees is
demonstrated.

Shoulder

The American Shoulder and Elbow Surgeons has agreed upon and adopted measuring shoulder motion as follows: elevation in the frontal plane, active and passive in degrees **(Figs. 4-23 and 4-24, respect.)**; external rotation with the arm at the side, active and passive in degrees; **(Figs. 4-25 and 4-26, respect.)**; internal rotation with the arm at the side, active or passive by where the hitchhiking thumb reaches in reference to posterior anatomy **(Fig. 4-27)**; external

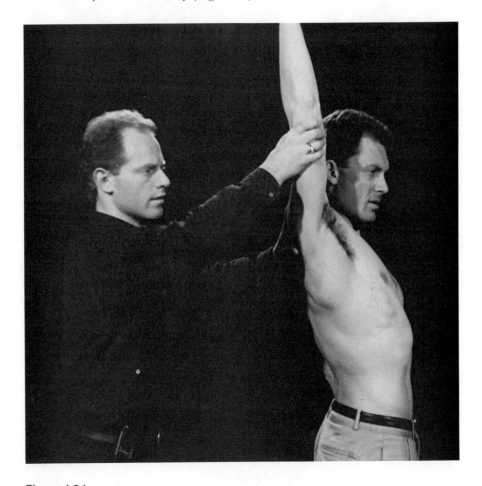

Figure 4-24.
The examiner is demonstrating passive elevation of the shoulder documented in degrees, taking into consideration the upper arm and the thorax. This patient has 180 degrees of passive elevation.

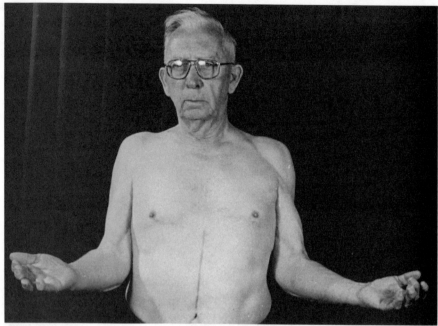

Figure 4-25.
Active external rotation is documented in degrees with the
arms comfortably at the sides.

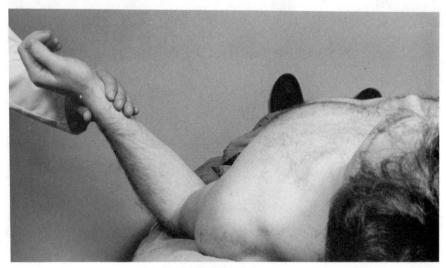

Figure 4-26.
Passive external rotation of the shoulder can be demonstrated in the supine position. This patient demonstrates 40
degrees of passive external rotation with the arm at the side
in the supine position.

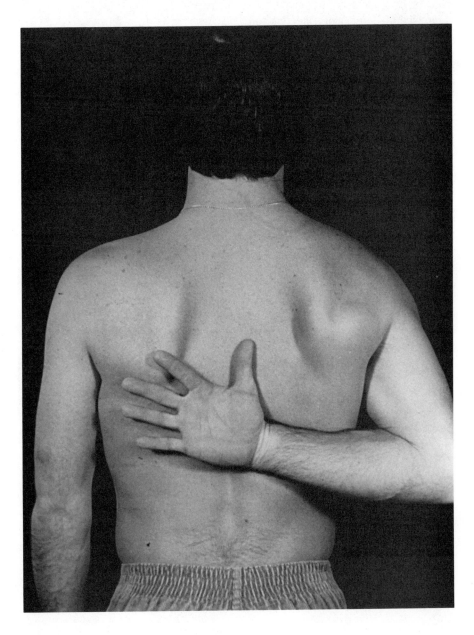

Figure 4-27.
Internal rotation is demonstrated by where the hitchhiking
thumb reaches in reference to spinous processes performed
either actively or passively.

rotation with the arm at the side and abducted to 90 degrees if 90 degrees of abduction can be achieved in increments (Fig. 4-28).

Interestingly, many normal patients have external rotation from 0 to 45 degrees with the arm at their side, whereas in the abducted position at 90 degrees normal patients have external rotation from 0 to 100 degrees. This difference relates to Codman's paradox and illustrates the confusion that exists when the arm is rotated in the abducted position.

External rotation in abduction is important in athletes, especially throwers (Fig. 4-29), those who have

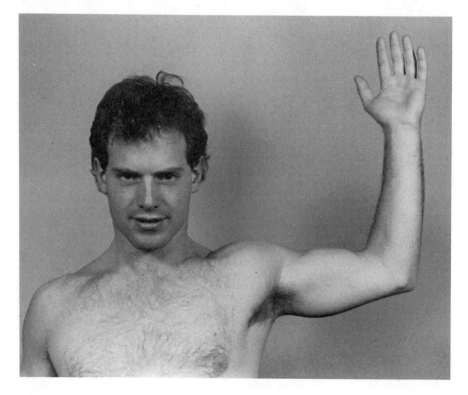

Figure 4-28.
External rotation is performed in the 90 degree abducted position and can be performed actively or passively. This can obviously be performed only if 90 degrees of abduction can be achieved. This patient demonstrates 90 degrees of external rotation in that position.

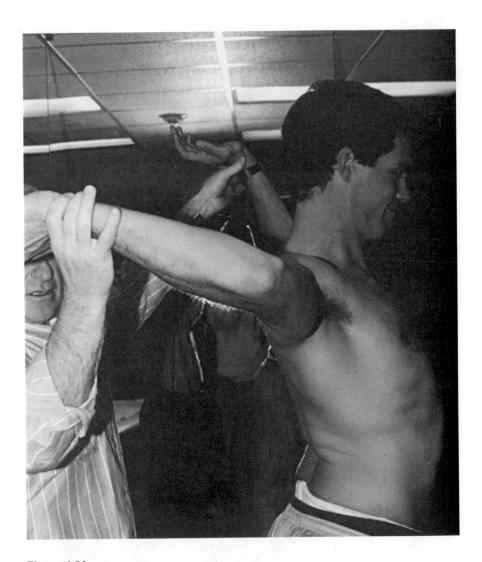

Figure 4-29.
Documentation of external rotation in the abducted position is very important in the athlete who is a thrower. This professional baseball player has excessive external rotation on the right arm, going to approximately 160 degrees in the 90 degree abducted position.

had a fracture, and those who have anterior instability with apprehension in this position **(Fig. 4-30)**.

Normally, no distinction is made between scapulothoracic versus glenohumeral contributions to motion; rather, the entire motion of the shoulder complex is examined and documented accordingly. Sometimes, however, isolating the role of each component is important. The scapulothoracic joint can be isolated by putting forefinger and thumb on the inferior border of the scapula and noting its contribution to overall motion **(Fig. 4-31, A, B)**. This is particularly applicable in patients with adhesive capsulitis.

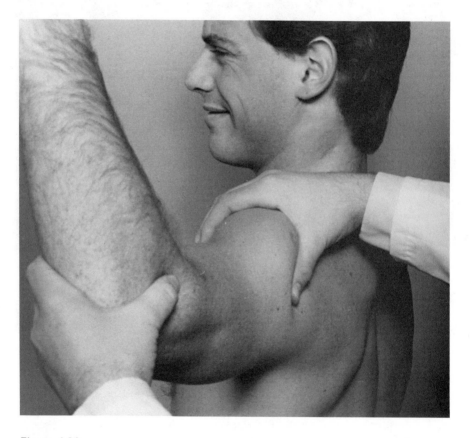

Figure 4-30.
Passive external rotation in the abducted position is also important in determining an apprehension sign, suggestive of anterior instability.

Many planes of motion in the shoulder are not documented on the chart either scientifically or by convention. For example, elevation in the sagittal plane, the frontal plane (**Fig. 4-9**), the scapular plane (**Fig. 4-32**), and in the coronal plane (**Fig. 4-33**) are not documented. Physicians do put shoulders through each of these motions to note differences and other physical features that may be present with these motions, for example, the presence of a painful arc with abduction in the coronal plane. The painful arc may be augmented with resistance (**Fig. 4-33**). Additionally, extension in many planes, such as the sagittal and horizontal planes, is often noted but not documented.

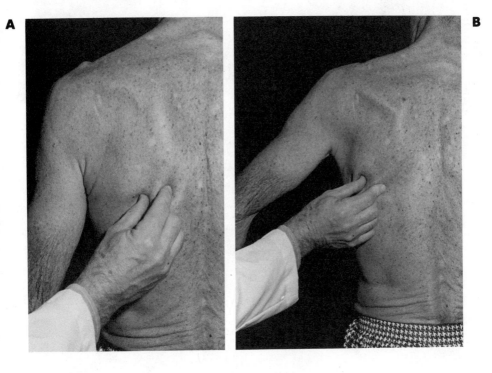

A

B

Figure 4-31.
A, B, The contribution of motion can be isolated from the scapulothoracic joint by putting the forefinger and thumb on the inferior border of the scapula and documenting its contribution to overall motion with elevation.

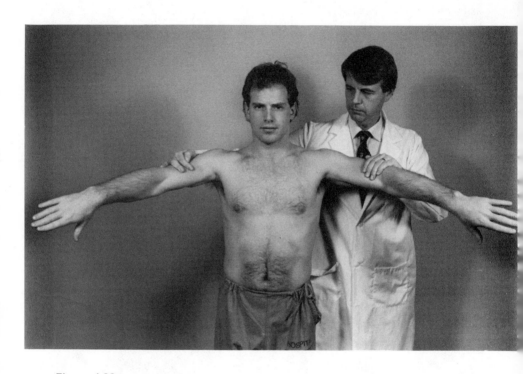

Figure 4-32.

This assesses elevation in the scapular plane, which is approximately 30 degrees anterior to the coronal plane. This patient is about to have strength tested in that position.

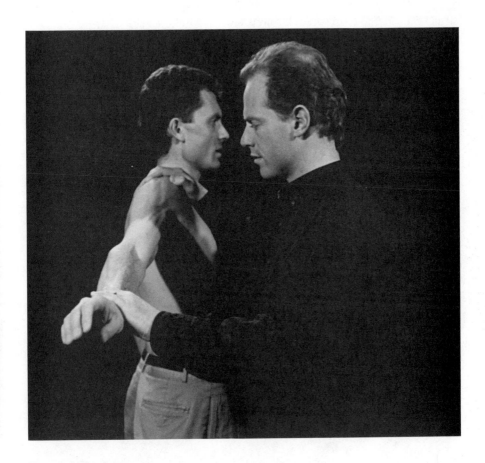

Figure 4-33.
Abduction occurs in the coronal plane and, along with
elevation and external rotation, is an important strength
measurement position.

Elbow

By convention, flexion **(Fig. 4-34)** and extension **(Fig. 4-35)** are measured in degrees beginning at zero. Supination **(Fig. 4-36)** and pronation are documented with the arm at the side, the elbow flexed to 90 degrees, and the shoulder in neutral rotation with the forearm straight ahead. The zero degree starting position is with the hitchhiking thumb pointing upward.

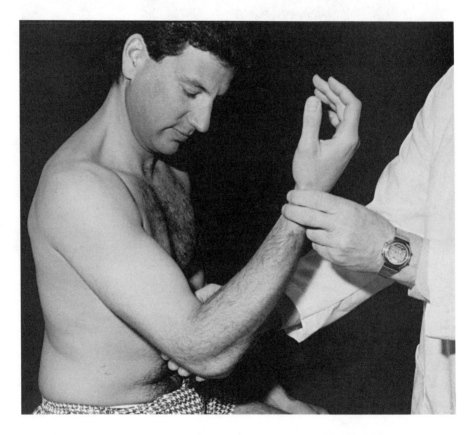

Figure 4-34.
Elbow flexion is determined actively and passively and documented in degrees, here at 95 degrees.

Figure 4-35.
Elbow extension is determined actively and passively and documented in degrees, here at 0 degrees.

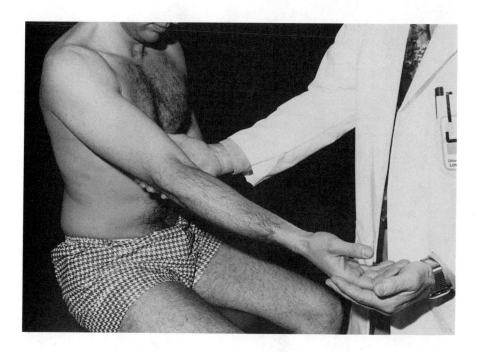

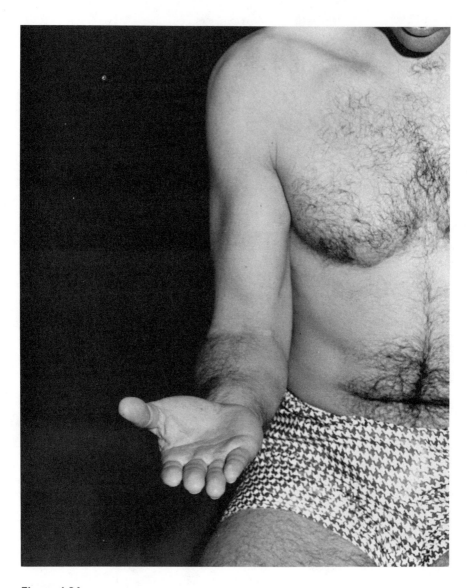

Figure 4-36.

Supination is documented with the arm comfortably at the side and turning the palm upward. This patient has full or 90 degrees of supination. Pronation is similarly documented.

Wrist

Wrist motion is measured in flexion described as either palmar or volar flexion **(Fig. 4-37)**, extension or dorsiflexion **(Fig. 4-38)**, both beginning at zero degrees or neutral, which is straight. At the wrist, radial **(Fig. 4-39)** and ulnar **(Fig. 4-40)** deviations are also documented, and are described as such to avoid the confusion of lateral and medial when the hand and wrist are supinated or pronated. Radial and ulnar deviation are documented in degrees relative to the midline.

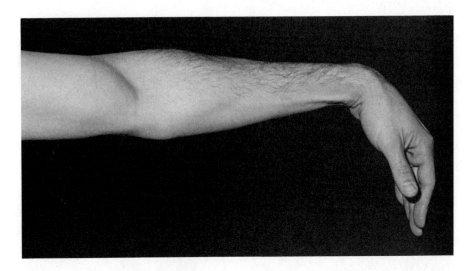

Figure 4-37.
Palmar flexion is documented in the wrist actively and passively. This patient demonstrates 70 degrees of palmar flexion.

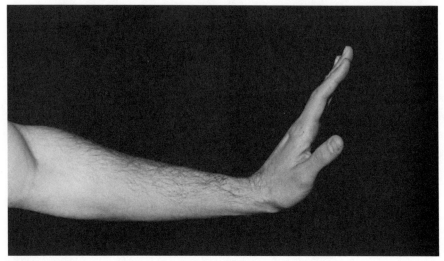

Figure 4-38.
Dorsiflexion is documented in the wrist actively and passively. This patient demonstrates 65 degrees of active dorsiflexion.

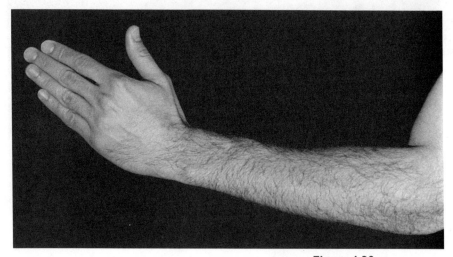

Figure 4-39.
Radial deviation is documented at the wrist in degrees. This patient demonstrates 30 degrees of radial deviation.

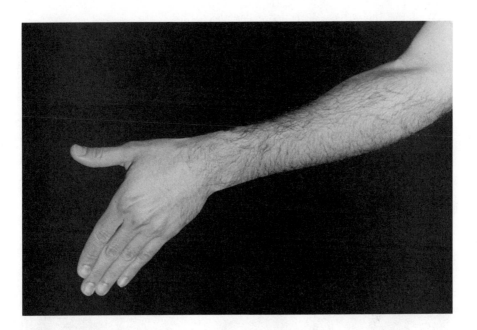

Figure 4-40.
Ulnar deviation is documented at the wrist in degrees. This patient demonstrates 35 degrees of ulnar deviation at the wrist.

Hand Joints

Each joint of the hand, which includes the thumb and all four fingers, is documented actively and passively beginning at neutral or zero degrees **(Fig. 4-15).** Flexion and extension of both the metacarpophalangeal joints are determined, as well as the proximal and distal interphalangeal joints of the fingers **(Fig. 4-41).** The metacarpal joint and the interphalangeal joint of the thumb are documented similarly. The carpometacarpal joint of the thumb is a little more complex, going through motions of flexion, extension, abduction, and adduction, in addition to abduction at right angles to the palm **(Fig. 4-42, A, B).**

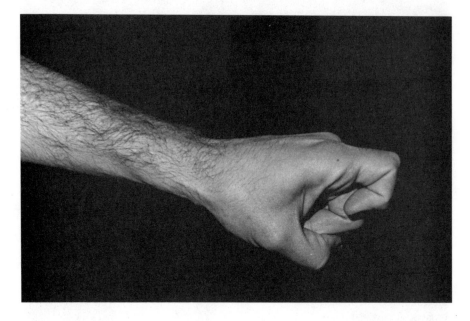

Figure 4-41.
Flexion of the proximal interphalangeal (PIP) and distal interphalangeal (DIP) joints are documented actively and passively. This patient demonstrates 110 degrees of active PIP flexion and 70 degrees of active DIP flexion.

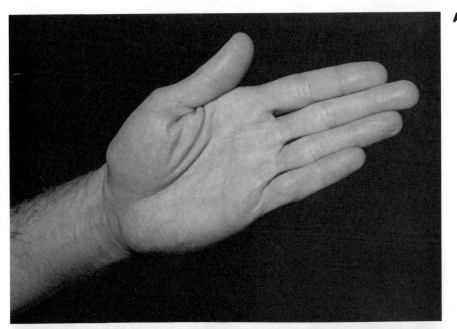

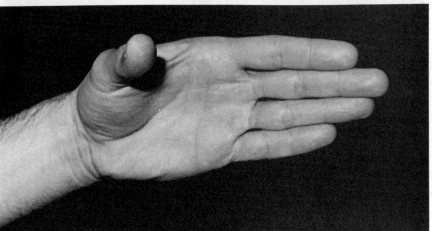

Figure 4-42.
A, B, Abduction of the thumb is documented at right angles to the plane of the hand. This patient is demonstrating adbduction of the thumb from 0 to 70 degrees.

Lumbar Spine

Documented spinal measurements are flexion relative to where the patient's hands reach in terms of the anatomy of the distal extremity or the floor if flat (Fig. 4-17), extension as a percentage of normal (Fig. 4-20), lateral flexion from the midline in degrees (Fig. 4-43), and rotation in degrees or an estimate from normal. Rotation is difficult to determine accurately because it is influenced by the entire spine and pelvis, and isolating the lumbar spine rotation is confusing (Fig. 4-44).

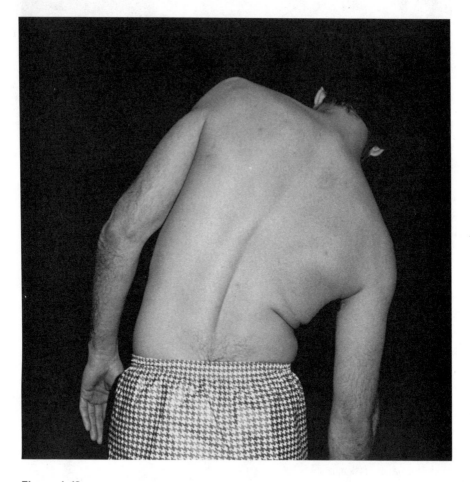

Figure 4-43.
Lateral flexion of the lumbar spine is determined by degrees from the midline.

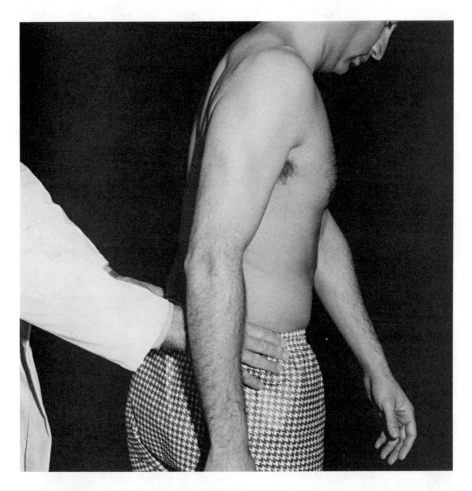

Figure 4-44.
Rotation of the lumbar spine is difficult to determine accurately because it is influenced by the entire spine and pelvis. Nevertheless, the rotation is documented as accurately as possible, in degrees, from the midline.

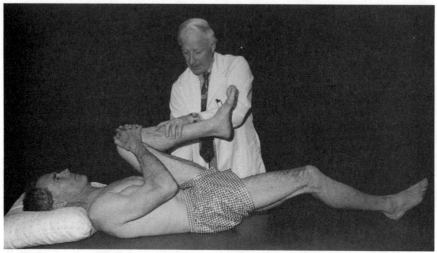

Figure 4-45.
The first part of the Thomas test for hip flexion is demonstrated, showing a 20-degree flexion deformity. A hand placed
behind the spine ensures a flat lumbar spine.

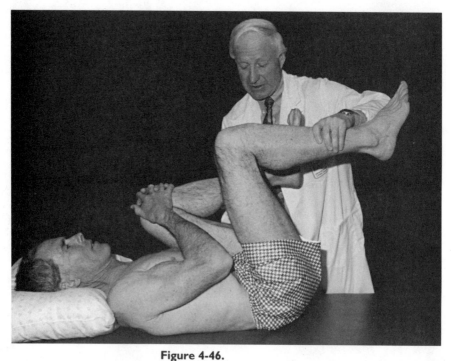

Figure 4-46.
The second part of the Thomas test, demonstrating flexion of
the right hip from its flexion deformity of 20 to 100 degrees
performed passively, is shown.

Hip

By convention, hip flexion **(Fig. 4-45)** and extension **(Fig. 4-46)** are documented in degrees; abduction and adduction in degrees with the pelvis placed at neutral; external and internal rotation in degrees, both in extension **(Fig. 4-47)** and at 90 degrees of flexion **(Fig. 4-48)**, using the sagittal plane as the midline. Extension of the hip is usually not measured, particularly because many patients with hip pathology have a flexion deformity **(Fig. 4-45)**. Hip motions are performed supine.

Knee

Documentation of knee measurements is in flexion **(Fig. 4-48)** and extension **(Fig. 4-3)**, both in degrees.

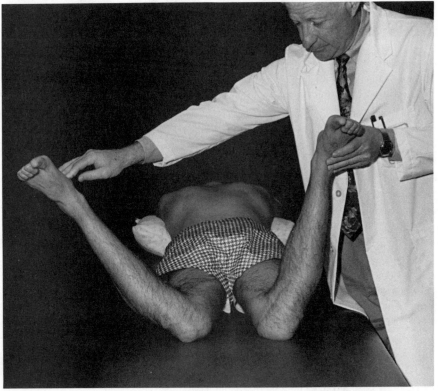

Figure 4-47.
External rotation of the hips in the prone position or in extension, is demonstrated.

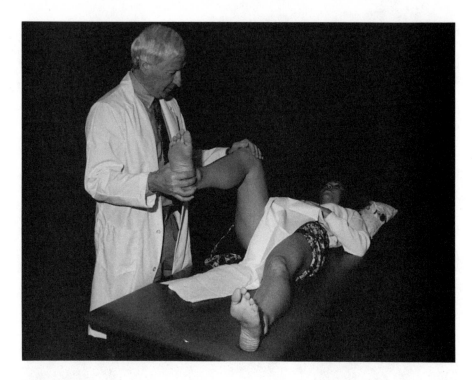

Figure 4-48.
External rotation of the hip in the supine position, using the
sagittal plane as the midline is demonstrated. Here the knee
is flexed to 90 degrees.

Ankle

Documenting the motions of the ankle is confusing
and the application of different terms is sometimes
misleading. This is because physicians often describe
both motions of the ankle and foot interchangeably and
confuse these motions with positions of the foot. Physicians document both plantar flexion **(Fig. 4-49, A)**
and extension **(Fig. 4-49, B)**, or dorsiflexion, in degrees, beginning at neutral or zero. The ankle also
moves in internal **(Fig. 4-49, C)** and external **(Fig.
4-49, D)** rotation, both measured in degrees.

Abduction **(Fig. 4-50, A)** and adduction **(Fig. 4-50,
B)**, or eversion and inversion, of the hindfoot related to
the ankle are sometimes documented, but contributions to these motions also come from the subtalar

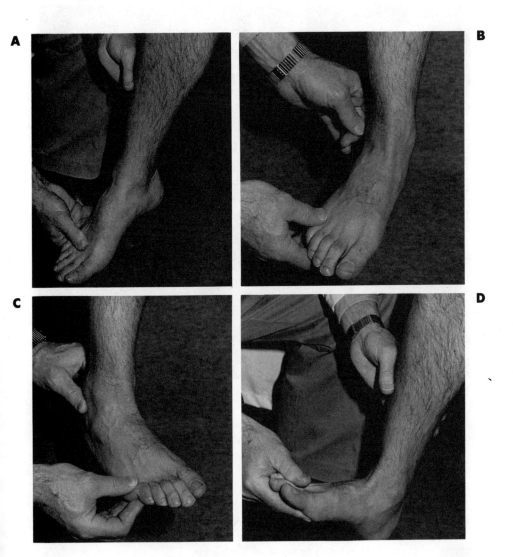

Figure 4-49.
A, Passive plantar flexion of the ankle to approximately 35 degrees is demonstrated. This motion is also documented actively. B, Passive dorsiflexion of the ankle to approximately 10 degrees is demonstrated. This motion is also documented actively. C, Internal rotation of the ankle passively to approximately 20 degrees is demonstrated. This motion is also documented actively. D, External rotation of the ankle passively to approximately 20 degrees is demonstrated. This motion is also documented actively.

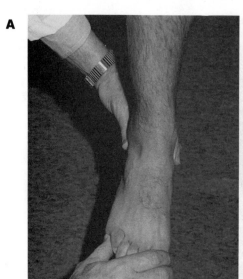

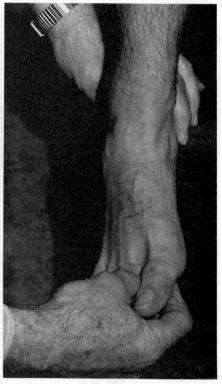

joint. At the subtalar joint, the measurement is passive, whereas in the ankle joint it is both active and passive. Varus and valgus of the hindfoot or heel are more often applied to describe positions rather than motions (Fig. 4-51).

Subtalar Joint

Measurements of subtalar motion are passive estimates at best and are difficult to separate from ankle motion.

Midtarsal Joint

Midtarsal joint motion consists of abduction and adduction, inversion and eversion, and rotation. These can be documented in degrees or estimates of normal and are best performed passively. Supination and pronation of the forefoot refer to positions rather than motions such as varus and valgus of the heel. Isolating midtarsal motions of the foot is difficult.

Figure 4-50.
A, Abduction of the ankle, which also describes a position of the foot, is demonstrated. B, Adduction of the ankle, which also describes a position of the foot, is demonstrated.

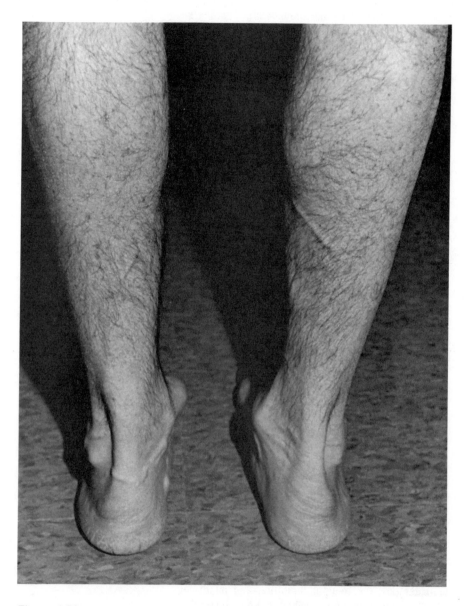

Figure 4-51.
Terms applied to the ankle and foot can be confusing.
Positions, such as *varus* and *valgus*, are commonly applied to
the foot. This patient demonstrates slight *valgus* deformities
of the hindfeet.

Toes

Motions of the toes are documented in degrees beginning at zero degrees, measuring metatarsophalangeal and interphalangeal joints.

Other Features of Joint Motions
Abnormal Motions

If a joint normally goes to zero degrees of extension and that is its limit, anything beyond that is referred to as abnormal motion and designated as such, for example, hyperextension or recurvatum of the knee. This might also occur in the distal interphalangeal joints of the fingers or the elbow joint.

If a joint such as the wrist normally goes beyond the neutral or zero position, it is not given an abnormal connotation but a positive connotation such as 60 degrees of extension or dorsiflexion of the wrist **(Fig. 4-39)**. This might also apply to the ankle or hip.

Active versus Passive Motion

A difference between active and passive motion might be due either to muscle deficiency, a neurological problem, or pain with its associated weakness.

Frequently, elderly patients who can elevate their shoulders actively 30 or 40 degrees and passively up to 170 degrees **(Fig. 4-52)** obviously have a significant problem, such as a rotator cuff tear. Rarely, however, such a patient may have much less common pathology, such as compression of the C5 root causing similar findings. A patient who presents with drop foot due to an L5 root lesion, may actively dorsiflex to neutral but passively can be dorsiflexed another 40 degrees related to the neurological deficiency. Likewise, a patient whose knee pain precludes him from performing active motion may achieve motion with support and coercion.

After knee surgery, the patient may have active extension to 15 degrees and passively may be taken to 0 degrees due to pain inhibition and quadriceps insufficiency. This is described as an *extensor* or *extension lag*.

Joint Deformities (Contractures)

Joint deformities play an important role with regard to active and passive ranges of motion. Joint deformities are determined by passive motion. Physicians may

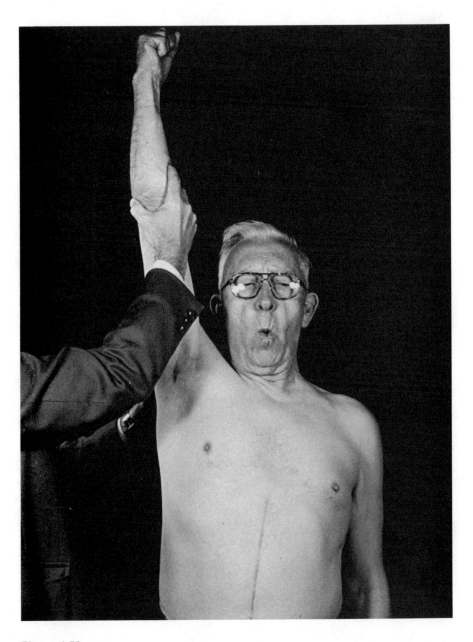

Figure 4-52.
Physicians frequently see elderly patients who can actively elevate their shoulders 30 to 40 degrees; passively they can be almost fully elevated, often with pain at this extreme (i.e., a sign of impingement).

reasonably use the term *deformity* until the specific cause of the deformity has been determined, be it soft tissue (*contracture*) or mechanical incongruency due to arthritis or intraarticular pathology, such as a meniscal tear. Determination of deformities is especially relevant to hip examination. The classical method of determining flexion deformities of the hip is with the Thomas test (**Fig. 4-53**). Such deformities are usually

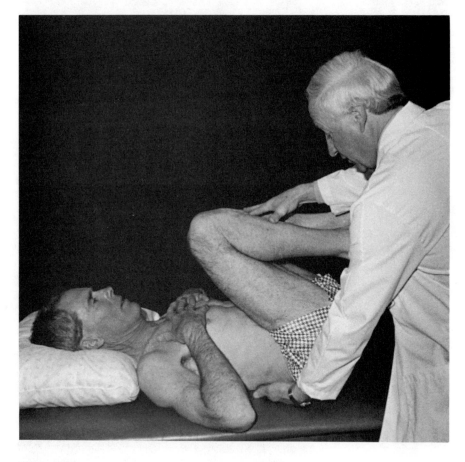

Figure 4-53.
The classical method of determining a flexion deformity of the hip is documented with the Thomas test. This figure demonstrates maximal flexion of both hips and knees and placement of a hand under the lumbar spine to ensure that it is flat against the table top.

due to a soft tissue contracture and are designated as such, for example, a 30 degree flexion contracture of the hip (**Fig. 4-54**). The range of motion must then be documented from that position, assessing the further range that may be present (**Fig. 4-46**). For example, in the presence of a flexion deformity of 20 degrees, the hip frequently will flex up to 90 degrees, giving an overall range of 70 degrees. In this situation, starting the range of motion at zero degrees of flexion would be inaccurate. The hip with this pathology does not even reach zero degrees. In documenting this on the chart, the examiner should write "hip flexion, 20 to 90 degrees," which implies a 20-degree flexion deformity and from there the hip flexes an additional 70 degrees up to 90 degrees. In this scenario, in the presence of a flexion deformity of the hip, documenting extension is obviously not necessary. In fact, with a hip examination, physicians normally do not document extension.

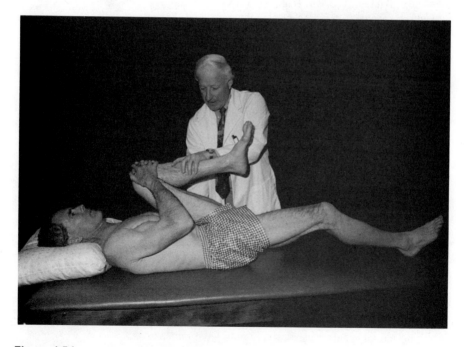

Figure 4-54.
From the previously demonstrated position, the left leg is held up maximally and the right leg brought down to the table top, indicating a 30 degree flexion deformity.

Other contractures or deformities applied to the hip include external rotation and adduction. If a deformity or contracture in one direction of motion (such as external rotation) exists and the part does not come back to neutral or zero, then under such circumstances the opposite motion (such as internal rotation) need not be documented because it cannot be achieved. Similarly, if a patient has a 20 degree adduction deformity of the right hip, the physician need not establish the amount of abduction. If the opposite motion were described, it would have a minus connotation. All of these principles can be applied to different joints in the body.

Determination of contractures are passive. With contractures, active motion usually equals passive motion, but that may not always be the situation. A patient may have a 20 degree flexion deformity in the knee but actively may be only able to extend to 30 degrees, leaving a 10 degree extension lag. A fixed deformity might be reserved to imply no motion, either actively or passively, in whatever plane is described. A knee fused at 10 degrees represents a fixed deformity. In the knee, some surgeons describe a block to extension as a *locked knee*.

Additional Features of Motion

During active and passive motion the physician must observe pain, rhythm, and crepitus.

Pain

Pain may occur throughout the range of motion (**Fig. 4-55**), only at the extremes of active motion (**Fig. 4-56**), or only when the part is stressed passively at the extremes of motion (**Fig. 4-52**). Sometimes the pain of active motion is diminished or eliminated when the part is supported and moved passively (**Fig. 4-57**). At the extremes of motion, all ranges should be stressed to elicit any pain that may be present. This may be a subtle positive physical finding, but it can be a reliable and important clinical sign (**Fig. 4-58**) because many early and mild pathological processes may only have pain when stressed at the extremes of motion; for example, eliciting pain when the hip is stressed with external rotation in the presence of a very early slipped capital femoral epiphysis.

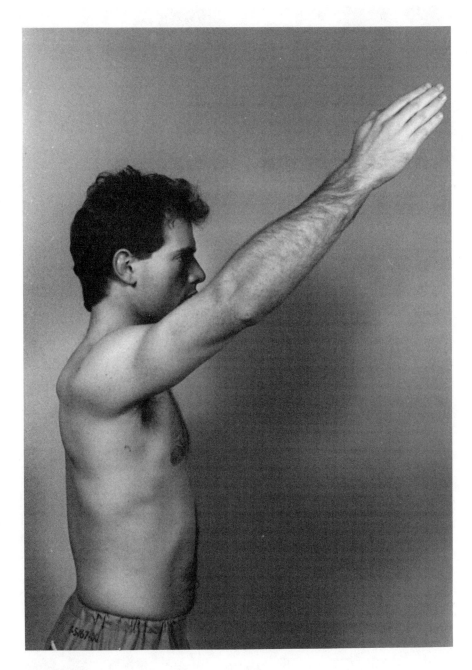

Figure 4-55.
Active elevation of a part can be painful throughout its range.

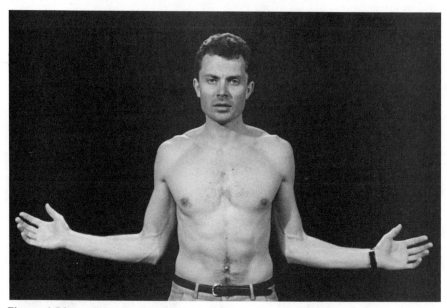

Figure 4-56.
Active range of motion may produce pain at the extremities of
motion.

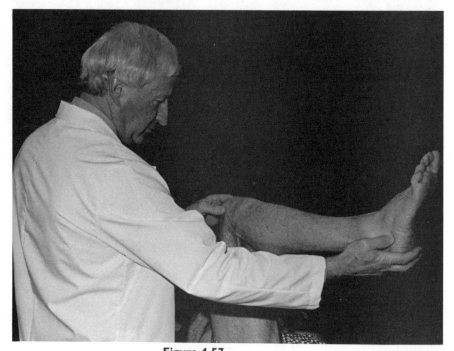

Figure 4-57.
Sometimes the pain of active motion is diminished or eliminated when the part is supported and moved only passively.

Rhythm

Documenting the rhythm or fluidity of motion may be meaningful. Rhythm may be influenced by pain, structural abnormalities, or neurological deficits. Patients who have a painful shoulder often avoid elevating into a painful position by moving the shoulder through various contortions. Patients who have a loose body in their knee may hesitate and move in a peculiar manner to avoid impinging this loose body between the condyles. Neurological diseases such as parkinsonism can also cause a part to move with abnormal rhythm.

As the patient with a rotator cuff tear elevates his shoulder, he may reach his destination in an abnormal fashion. This may be due either to weakness in certain ranges or to impingement of the tendons under the acromion. Patients with subacromial scarring related to a rotator cuff tear frequently grasp their arm for

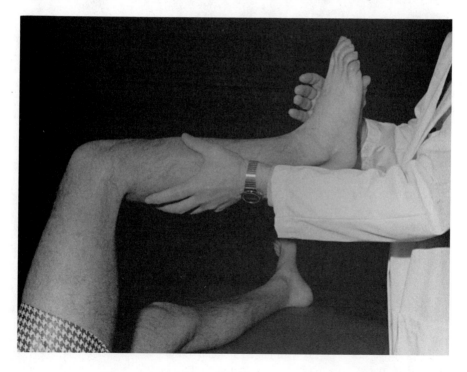

Figure 4-58.
Pain with stressed external rotation of the hip may suggest the presence of a very early slipped capital femoral epiphysis.

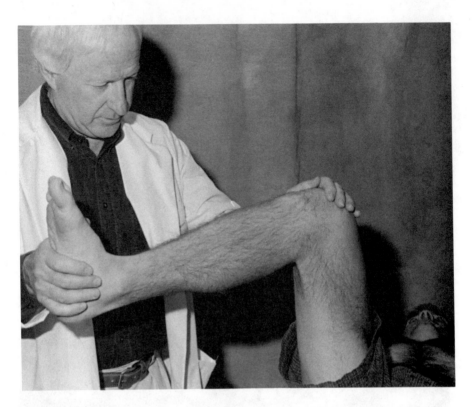

Figure 4-59.
In a hip with a slipped capital femoral epiphysis, flexion often occurs only in an externally rotated plane. This is known as a Howorth sign and represents an unusual plane of motion.

support when lowering the arm and shoulder from an elevated position. Occasionally, an abnormal or unusual plane of motion is present. For example, in a hip with a slipped capital femoral epiphysis, flexion may only occur with external rotation; this is known as a Howorth sign **(Fig. 4-59)**.

Crepitus

The presence or absence of crepitus may be associated with certain diagnoses. Crepitus may be felt or heard. It may be palpated over the part being examined with passive or active motion, and it may be of a soft tissue or a bony nature. Bone crepitus from osteoarthritis has a much harsher characteristic than the quieter crepitus related to soft tissue scarring. Patients who have patellar crepitus with knee extension often have a palpable bone-on-bone feel to the crepitus, frequently determined actively and sometimes passively. The best method for determining patellar crepitus is by placing a hand on the patella of the patient, who is seated, and having the patient actively extend the knee (**Fig. 4-60**). Perhaps the best way to elicit crepitus in the subacromial bursa is with passive rotation of the shoulder. Painful crepitus of the shoulder with passive rotation in the abducted position may

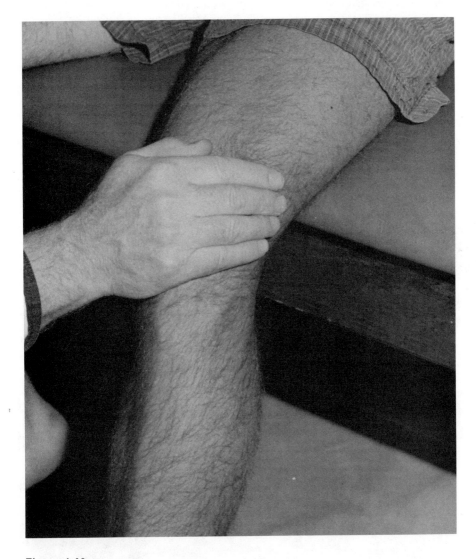

Figure 4-60.
The best method to determine patellar crepitus is having the patient, while seated, actively extend the lower extremity with the examiner's hand placed over the patella.

suggest impingement tendonitis, which is common with a cuff tear. With resisted elevation of the shoulder to approximately 90 degrees, a fairly obvious crunching of the shoulder emanating from bone-on-bone crepitus due to osteoarthritis may occur. Similarly, passive motion occurring with simple rotation of the arm at the side may be present in patients who have a rotator cuff deficiency and is much softer. Palpable crepitus with direct pressure is unusual, but may occur over the synovium in patients with rheumatoid arthritis, gas gangrene, or subcutaneous emphysema.

Figure 4-61.
While putting the knee through a range of motion, assessing quadriceps strength at this stage is appropriate.

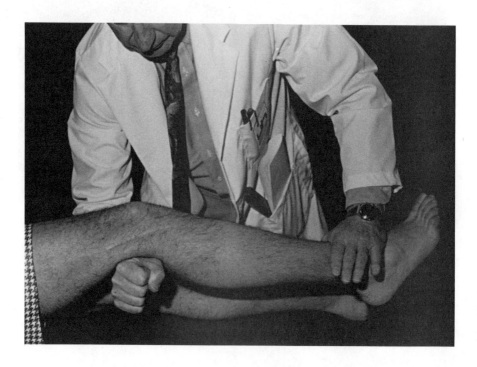

Neurological Strength Testing

While the patient is demonstrating active range of motion, applying resistance and determining a grade of strength using the classical Medical Research Council 0 to 5 rating system (Table 4-2) seems appropriate. The logical time to assess quadriceps strength is as the patient demonstrates active flexion and extension of the knee (Fig. 4-61). Strength is determined isometrically, represented by the maximal exertion performed against resistance and is compared to the opposite side.

TABLE 4-2
GRADING OF MUSCLE STRENGTH USING THE MEDICAL RESEARCH COUNCIL 0-5 RATING SYSTEM

Grade	Degree of Muscle Strength	Descriptive Term
0 = Zero	No palpable contraction	Nothing
1 = Trace	Muscle contracts, but part normally motorized does not move	Trace
2 = Poor	Muscle moves the part but not against gravity	With gravity eliminated
3 = Fair	Muscle moves part through a range against gravity	Against gravity
4 = Good	Muscle moves part even against added resistance; variations in resistance graded plus or minus	Near normal
5 = Excellent	Normal strength against resistance is present	Normal

Principles of Muscle Testing

When testing strength, a reproducible technique that takes into consideration the factors that may influence an accurate estimate of strength is needed. The following guidelines should be used to assess strength during the physical examination.

1. The individual muscle to be assessed should be given the mechanical advantage (Fig. 4-62). This may be accomplished by appropriate positioning of the joint; for example, testing elbow flexion is most reliably performed at 90 degrees.

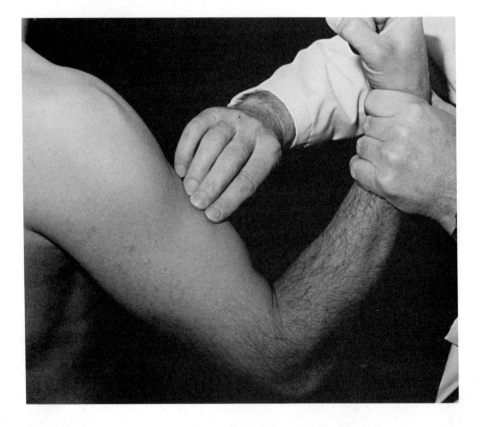

Figure 4-62.
The muscles to be tested should be given the mechanical advantage. The bicep muscle or elbow flexion is maximally efficient at 90 degrees of flexion. The examiner should always attempt to visually observe and palpate the contracting muscle.

2. After the limb is appropriately positioned, the examiner should always attempt to feel and to see the muscle contraction **(Fig. 4-62).**

3. When testing muscle groups, the strength rating may vary throughout the arc of movement because of the recruitment of different muscles. Hence the strength rating must be broken down into the component parts of the arc; for example, abduction at 90 degrees may be more powerful than abduction at the side and reflects more muscles working at a better mechanical advantage **(Fig. 4-63).**

4. Gradual resistance should be applied and a grade ranging from 0 to 5 assigned. Sometimes at the higher grades, (e.g., 3 or 4), the addition of plusses or minuses indicates more subtle variations.

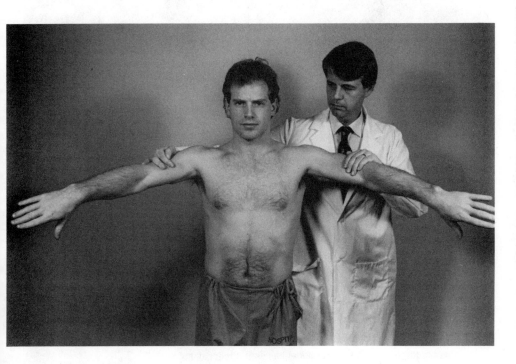

Figure 4-63.
Abduction at 90 degrees may be more powerful than abduction at the side and reflects a better mechanical advantage.

5. If the opposite side is normal, strength should be compared to it. In a bodybuilder, for example, subtle weakness may be missed if the muscle power is compared to another patient with average strength.

6. In the presence of significant pain, recording muscle strength may be unreliable unless a painless arc can be found **(Figs. 4-64, 4-65)**.

Examiners sometimes assess gross movement of a joint provided by several muscles such as hip flexion,

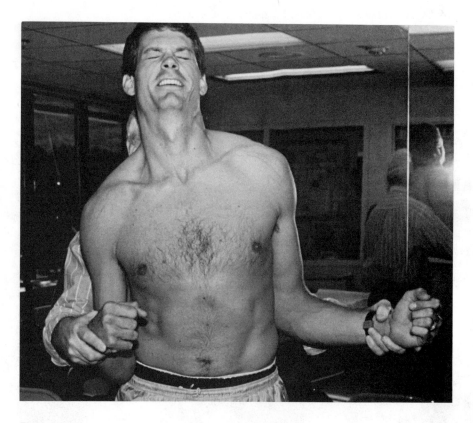

Figure 4-64.
In the presence of significant pain, recording muscle strength may be unreliable. This professional baseball pitcher demonstrates significant pain with resisted external rotation of the right arm. Whether this represents true weakness is yet to be determined.

and they sometimes assess a simple movement provided by one muscle such as the first dorsal interosseous (Fig. 4-66). Obviously the overlapping nerve supply is related to central root innervation versus peripheral innervation, which must be considered as motions and strength are analyzed.

In performing resistance testing of elbow flexion, the elbow flexors, particularly the brachialis, should be at a mechanical advantage, which is at approximately 90 degrees of flexion (Fig. 4-62). This principle of allowing the part the mechanical advantage applies to most muscle groups in most circumstances. Occasionally, however, taking the advantage away would be helpful because grading differences between 4 and 5 may prove difficult. This would apply to a 300-pound lineman when assessing his quadriceps, in that grade 4 could be interpreted as normal. In this circumstance, rather than allowing the quadriceps the mechanical advantage in extension, one should have the patient flex

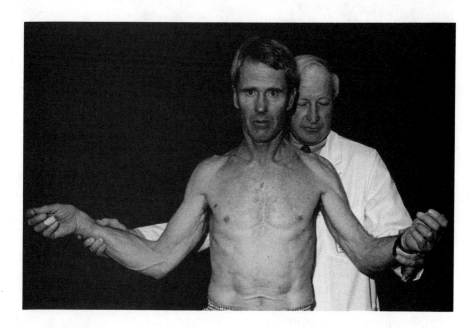

Figure 4-65.
If pain is present, assessing muscle strength in as pain free a range as can be found may result in a more meaningful examination.

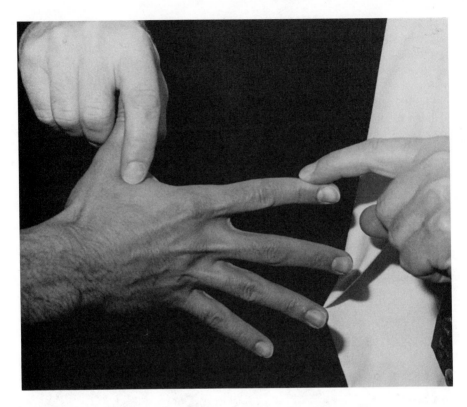

Figure 4-66.
Sometimes physicians assess simple movements supplied by one muscle, such as abduction of the index finger provided by the first dorsal interosseous muscle. The contraction is palpated and visualized.

the knee and then apply resistance to get a more subtle reading of weakness. Even mere visual inspection and palpation of the bulk and contour of a muscular contraction may suggest that it is normal **(Figs. 4-62, 4-66)**.

As stated, a full range of motion of the part is necessary before muscle strength rating can be entertained. Obviously, however, strength rating may vary throughout the range of a joint. For example, active elevation of the shoulder from 0 to 30 degrees may have Grade 4 muscle strength, whereas motion from 30 to 170 degrees may have Grade 2 muscle strength. If such a situation is present, the strength should be separately described by breaking it down into its component parts.

Within the system frequent liberties are taken by describing plusses and minuses. This is applicable, especially to Grade 4, because this grade is frequently inadequate to describe the variations in weakness that can occur. Physicians and therapists therefore frequently describe 4+ (plus) or 4– (minus). The presence of pain frequently confuses the issue and does not permit an accurate grading of muscle strength. Whether this rating system can even be employed in the presence of pain, however, is questionable. To aid in a more reliable determination, the part may be assessed in a range that is not painful. Often, the examiner can determine the presence of true weakness, even when pain is present. If not, the patient may have opinions as to whether he is truly weak.

In summary, the following principles apply to muscle testing:

1. The muscle to be assessed should be given the mechanical advantage.

2. The physician should feel and observe the muscle during testing.

3. Because strength may vary through an arc of movement, strength rating may need to be related to a specific arc.

4. Resistance should be applied gradually and assigned a grade (0 to 5).

5. The opposite, normal side should be used for comparison.

6. In the presence of significant pain, muscle strength recording may be inaccurate.

The previous aspects of muscle testing described herein apply not only to muscle strength, which comes under range of motion, but also to neurological examination consisting of the motor assessment, which is discussed in the subsequent chapter. Strength assessment therefore overlaps both mechanical assessment and neurological assessment. Frequently, in the postoperative stage, patients who have pain have weakness that is usually not due to a neurological deficiency but, rather, to pain. Some physicians (such as neurologists) prefer to leave this main part, that is, the neurological examination, to the end so that it receives a more direct focus. As part of the musculoskeletal approach, perhaps it is more appropriately positioned here to fit within the scheme. Because strength testing was done as part of range of motion representing the motor aspect, it can serve as the beginning of the neurological examination.

Chapter

5   Neurological Examination

The neurological examination is modified according to the patient's complaint, history, associated disease, general well-being, and the suspected or possible diagnosis. The physician should rule out a neurological cause for a patient's musculoskeletal complaint and should document any associated neurological findings indicating any diseases that may be present. Certain complaints and musculoskeletal findings may indicate the need for an extensive or general neurological assessment. Dividing the neurological examination into several components allows rapid assessment of potential pathology and is generally required to assess motor, sensory, reflex, and cerebellar functions. The presence of any upper motor neuron signs should be noted. The significance of documenting neurological function, particularly distal to an acute musculoskeletal lesion cannot be overemphasized. The status of the radial nerve in a patient with a humeral shaft fracture or the presence of a cervical spinal cord syndrome secondary to cervical spine fracture must be documented. How brief or extensive the neurological examination should be varies significantly. With examination of the musculoskeletal system, common sense dictates the appropriate degree of neurological assessment. Several examples best illustrate the variation in neurological presentation that can occur in different situations.

- A five-year-old patient who lacerates the tip of a finger should have a sensory and motor examination distal to the cut.
- A ten-year-old patient with hemiparesis should have stereognosis assessed prior to contemplating hand surgery.
- A 20-year-old patient with knee instability suggests neurological assessment distal to the level of the lesion.
- A 50-year-old patient with left hip and leg pain

requires an extensive neurological examination of
the lower extremities and perhaps even the upper
extremities along with testing for cerebellar abnormalities.

- A patient with right shoulder pain and weakness
  needs a thorough neurological examination of the
  upper extremities because of the differential diagnosis involving cervical spine versus shoulder and
  may even require examination of the lower extremities, noting in particular any upper motor
  neuron signs.

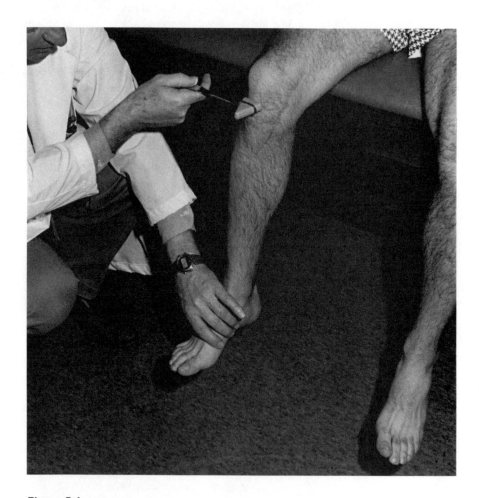

Figure 5-1.
Increased spasticity is manifest by hyperflexia and perhaps
most easily determined by examining the knee jerk reflex.

- A patient with rheumatoid arthritis who presents for metacarpophalangeal implants in the hand must have a thorough neurological examination of both upper and lower extremities, noting in particular the presence of upper motor neuron signs in the lower extremities consistent with spinal cord compression secondary to atlantoaxial instability. These consist of any evidence of increased tone such as increased spasticity (Fig. 5-1), sustained clonus (Fig. 5-2), or upgoing toes (Fig. 5-3). Although the examiner may choose to do little about this pathology, when using general anesthesia and endotracheal intubation, the anesthesiologist must be alerted to the presence of spinal cord compression from atlantoaxial instability.

In performing a neurological examination, the physician must keep in mind the distinction, yet overlap, between root and peripheral nerve innervation. Numbness in the index finger with associated dullness to pinprick may emanate from a median nerve compression in the carpal tunnel or a sixth cervical root compression. Additional features of history and physi-

Figure 5-2.
Sustained clonus of more than four beats is a manifestation of an upper motor neuron lesion.

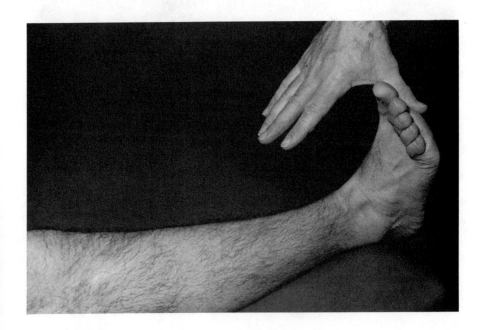

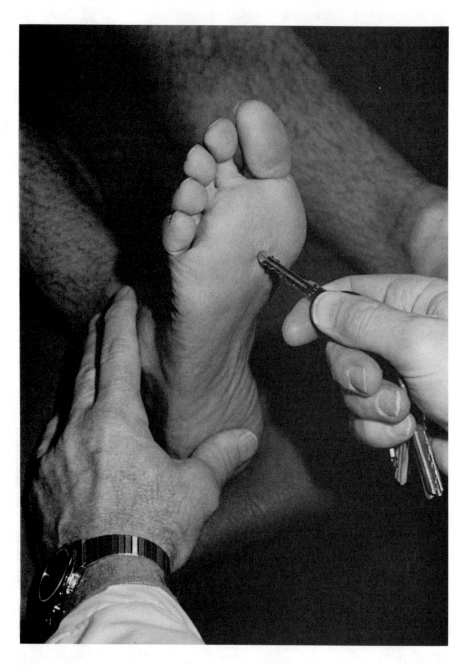

Figure 5-3.
Upgoing toes, previously termed a positive Babinski response, is suggestive of an upper motor neuron lesion.

cal examination probably will determine the area responsible.

In analyzing the neurological status of the patient, the examiner must consider strength, sensation, and reflexes among other signs that are relevant to the complaint and suspected diagnosis of the patient's problem. The method of assessing strength has already been described under the chapter on Range of Motion. Sensation consists of response to pinprick compared with the opposite side **(Fig. 5-4)**. Light touch might also be considered **(Fig. 5-5)**. For patients who have deficiencies in and about the hand, two-point discrimination is a more meaningful and reliable method of analyzing sensation **(Fig. 5-6)**. Reflexes are objective

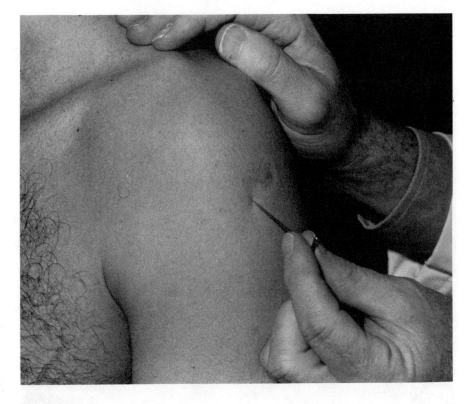

Figure 5-4.
Sensation is most commonly assessed by response to a pinprick compared with the opposite side. This patient demonstrates dullness to pinprick over the lateral aspect of the deltoid.

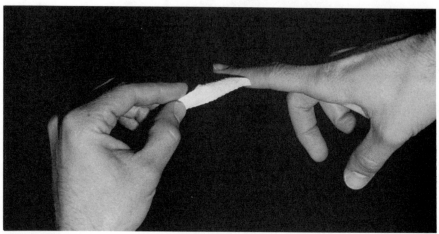

Figure 5-5.
Superficial sensation can also be determined by light touch and compared with the opposite side, but it is not as accurate and reliable as a pinprick.

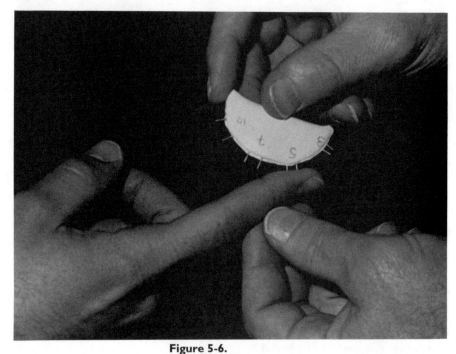

Figure 5-6.
Two-point discrimination is particularly meaningful and reliable in analyzing sensation, especially in the presence of peripheral nerve lesions.

and, as such, compared to strength and sensation, may be the most reliable of these neurological signs (Figs. 5-1, 5-7). Unfortunately, strength and sensation are influenced by subjective factors. Cerebellar assessment and balance can be important considerations in patients who have musculoskeletal disease.

The kind of speech should be reported; for example, whether dysphasia or dysarthria exists. If findings are positive, mention should be made as to the presence of auditory, visual, or tactile agnosia. Here, too, reference to spine motion, especially cervical spine motion, in

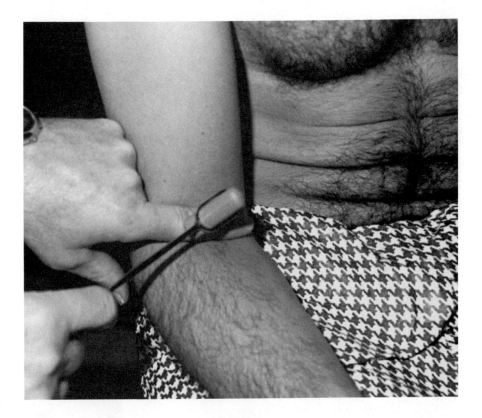

Figure 5-7.
The biceps reflex is determined by having the elbow flexed to approximately 90 degrees and relaxed in the patient's lap. The thumb is placed over the biceps tendon and gently tapped with the hammer. The elbow often flexes in the presence of a biceps contraction. The logical cervical route is C5, some C6. Comparison to the opposite side is necessary.

relationship to any neurological changes should be made. The examiner should be certain that during any portion of the medical examination harm is not done. For example, when a patient has a suspected fracture of the cervical spine, movement of the neck must be carefully performed or avoided altogether until a cross-table lateral x-ray is obtained. This is one of the few times the examiner must rely on excellent roentgeno-grams of the cervical spine before a comprehensive examination in order to establish a precise diagnosis of an injured part. If indicated, a thorough examination of the cranial and peripheral nervous system should be made.

If a patient is unconscious, confused, or drowsy, the physician's diagnostic skill is exceptionally important. The unconscious patient cannot relate a history or follow commands. A confused patient is disoriented, while a drowsy patient may be able to respond to verbal stimuli. Certain essential tests may be needed for unconscious patients, such as computed tomography for a space-occupying lesion. Young children and in-fants also fall into this category because a history cannot be communicated directly and so the physician must rely on specialized observational skills during the examination.

The examiner must bear in mind at all times the segmental supply of the muscles being examined re-lated to their peripheral nerve supply. Similarly, the examiner will find that knowing the sensory der-matomes of the skin is useful. Superficial sensation is tested by pinprick, (Fig. 5-4), while deep pain may be tested by squeezing the muscles of the limb. If indi-cated, vibration and cortical sensation should be tested. Two-point discrimination tests the ability of the patient to discriminate between two points (Fig. 5-6) and provides a more discriminating and subtle appre-ciation of superficial sensation. The physician should remember that the spinal cord is shorter than the vertebral column and terminates at the first lumbar vertebral level. The C8 spinal segment is opposite the seventh vertebrae, and L5 spinal segment exits the foramen between the L4 and L5 vertebrae.

The tendon reflexes, involuntary contractions of a muscle in response to a brisk tap on a tendon (Figs. 5-1, 5-7), can be divided into *deep* and *superficial.* For

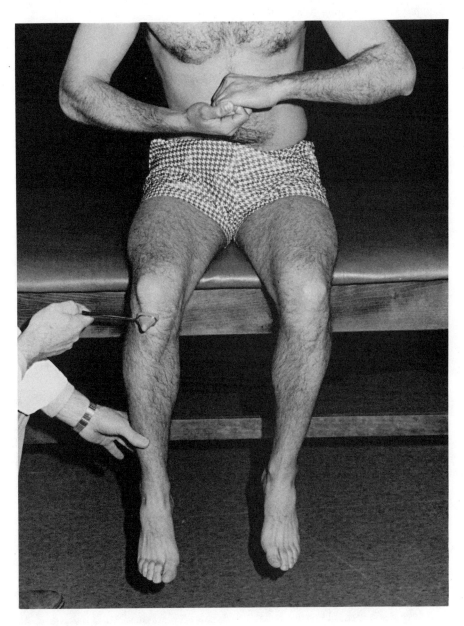

Figure 5-8.
This demonstrates the method of augmentation known as Jendrassik's maneuver, which can be performed when the knee reflex is difficult to elicit. The patient is asked to cup the hands, locking the fingers of both hands, and pull in opposite directions while the examiner taps the patellar tendon.

example, a deep tendon reflex such as the knee jerk depends upon the reflex contraction of the quadriceps and its central segmental innervation of L3-L4 supplied by the peripheral femoral nerve. A reflex may be absent and is termed 0; diminished, or rated as 1; average as 2; exaggerated as 3; or show clonus for a rating of 4. The reflexes on both sides of the body should be tested and

A

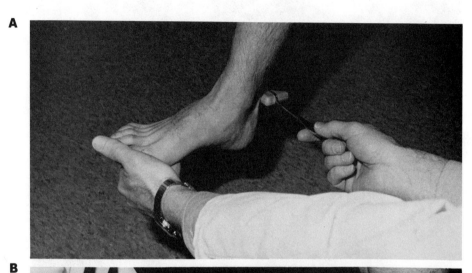

B

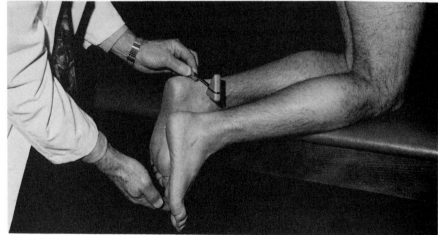

Figure 5-9.
A, The ankle reflex can be augmented when it is weak by asking the patient to plantarflex with slight pressure. B, The ankle reflex can be augmented by having the patient kneel on the examining table and then tapping the Achilles tendon.

compared. If a reflex is difficult to elicit, the test can often be performed by using reinforcement. In the lower extremity, Jendrassik's maneuver is used when the patient holds the hands together by cupping and locking the fingers of both hands and pulling in opposite directions (Fig. 5-8). The ankle reflex can be augmented by asking the patient to minimally contract into plantar flexion or having the patient kneel (Fig. 5-9, A, B). For the upper extremity, the same type of reinforcement may be achieved by clenching the hand not being examined or by biting hard. Abnormal reflexes such as the Babinski, which is now termed *upgoing toes*, should be considered if any suspicion of an upper motor neuron lesion exists (see Fig. 3-4). Primitive reflexes are normally demonstrated in early infancy and their early absence or manifestation at a later time can be of clinical significance. The Moro embrace reflex is present at birth until several months of age (Fig. 5-10)

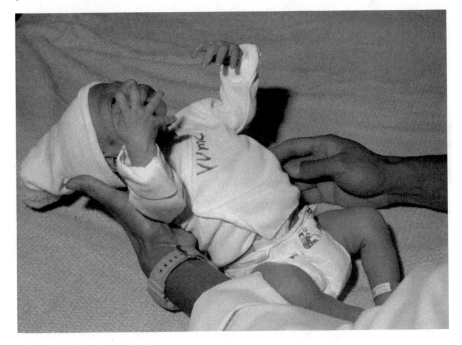

Figure 5-10.
The Moro embrace reflex is present at birth until several months of age. It may be absent early on in the presence of neurological disease, but may indicate cerebral disease if persistent after six months.

but may be absent on one side in the presence of a lower motor neuron lesion. If it is persistent after six months of age, it may indicate cerebral disease. A brachial plexus palsy or even a fractured clavicle at birth may show an absent Moro embrace reflex.

A neurological examination may be cursory or, if suggested by the patient's complaint, may be rather extensive. With a patient who has had a significant injury to the neck and shoulder area, the probability of a brachial plexus lesion requires an extensive neurological examination. In this situation, the physician should analyze weakness about the shoulder girdle, the proximal and distal upper extremity, as well as sensory and reflex changes, requiring a detailed examination. This helps localize the degree of brachial plexus lesion as well as its level. For such an examination, the physician may have to refer to standard textbooks for elaboration regarding such extensive neurological assessment.

Neurological Examination of Upper Limbs

The neurological examination of the upper limbs includes detailed muscle testing to define radicular or

Text continued on p. 157.

TABLE 5-1
NEUROLOGICAL ROOT LEVELS IN THE UPPER LIMB AND NECK

Level	Motor	Sensory	Reflex
C5	Deltoid biceps (partial)	Lateral deltoid	Biceps
C6	Biceps ECRL and ECRB	Thumb	Brachioradialis biceps
C7	Triceps wrist flexors finger extension	Middle finger	Triceps
C8	Finger flexors	Ulnar border little finger	—
T1	Intrinsics	Medial side proximal arm	—

ECRL, *Extensor carpi radialis longus;* ECRB, *extensor carpi radialis brevis.*

TABLE 5-2
MUSCLE TESTING CHART FOR UPPER EXTREMITIES

Muscle	Innervation (Peripheral Nerve)	Myotomes (Roots)	Technique for Testing
Biceps brachii	Musculocutaneous	C5-C6	Flexion of supinated forearm against resistance
Brachialis	Musculocutaneous	C5-C6	Resist flexion at elbow
Extensor carpi radialis longus	Radial	C5-C6	Resist wrist extension
Extensor carpi radialis brevis	Radial	C5-C7	Resist wrist extension
Extensor carpi ulnaris	Radial	C6-C8	Resist wrist extension
Extensor digitorum communis	Radial	C6-C8	Resist finger extension
Extensor indicis	Radial	C6-C8	Resist second finger extension
Extensor indicis minimi	Radial	C6-C8	Resist extension little finger
Brachioradialis	Radial	C5-C6	With forearm in neutral rotation and the elbow flexed 90 degrees against resistance, the contracting muscle is seen and palpated
Triceps	Radial	C5-C6	Resistance against extended elbow
Pronator teres	Median	C6-C7	On pronation of forearm against resistance, contraction of pronator teres palpated

Continued.

TABLE 5-2
MUSCLE TESTING CHART FOR
UPPER EXTREMITIES – cont'd.

Muscle	Innervation (Peripheral Nerve)	Myotomes (Roots)	Technique for Testing
Flexor carpi radialis	Median	C7-C8	Resist wrist flexion, abduction against closed hand
Flexor carpi ulnaris	Ulnar	C7-C8	Resist wrist flexion, adduction against closed hand
Flexor digitorum superficialis	Median	C7-C8	Stabilize fingers in flexion while resisting attempt to straighten fingers
Flexor digitorum profundus	Median (radial half) Ulnar (radial half)	C7-T1 C7-T1	Same test as noted above
Dorsal interossei	Ulnar	C8-T1	Resist finger abduction
Palmar interossei	Ulnar	C8-T1	Resist finger abduction
Abductor digiti quinti	Ulnar	C8-T1	Resist fifth finger abduction
Lumbricales (digits 1, 2)	Median	C7-T1	Resist MP and IP joint extension
Abductor pollicis brevis	Median	C8-T1	Resist thumb abduction
Opponens pollicis	Median	C8-T1	Resist opposition of thumb
Opponens digiti quinti	Ulnar	C8-T1	Same test as noted above

*MP, *Metacarpophalangeal;* IP, *interphalangeal.*

TABLE 5-3
MUSCLE TESTING CHART FOR SHOULDER

Muscle	Innervation (Peripheral Nerve)	Myotomes (Roots)	Technique for Testing
Trapezius	Spinal accessory	C2-C4	Patient shrugs shoulders against resistance
Sternomastoid	Spinal accessory	C2-C4	Patient turns head to one side with resistance over opposite temporal area
Serratus anterior	Long thoracic	C5-C7	Patient pushes against wall with outstretched arm, scapular winging is observed
Latissimus dorsi	Thoracodorsal	C7-C8	Downward/backward pressure of arm against resistance; muscle palpable at inferior angle of scapula during cough
Rhomboid	Dorsal	(C4)C5*	Hands on hips pushing elbows backward against resistance
Subclavius	N. to subcl.	C5-C6	None
Teres major	Subscapular (lower)	C5,C6	Similar to latissimus dorsi muscle palpable at lower border of scapula
Deltoid	Axillary	C5	With arm abducted 90 degrees downward pressure is applied; anterior and posterior fibers may be tested in slight flexion and extension
Subscapularis	Subscapular (upper)	C5	Arm at side with elbow flexed at 90 degrees; examiner resists internal rotation

Continued.

TABLE 5-3
MUSCLE TESTING CHART FOR SHOULDER – cont'd.

Muscle	Innervation (Peripheral Nerve)	Myotomes (Roots)	Technique for Testing
Supraspinatus	Suprascapular	C5(6)	Arm abducted against resistance (not isolated); with arm pronated and elevated 90 degrees in plane of scapula; downward pressure is applied
Infraspinatus	Suprascapular	C5(C6)	Arm at side with elbow flexed 90 degrees; examiner resists external rotation
Teres minor	Axillary	C5	Same as for infraspinatus
Pectoralis major	Medial and lateral pectoral	C5-T1	With arm flexed 30 degrees in front of body, patient adducts against resistance
Pectoralis minor	Medial pectoral	C8,T1	None
Coracobrachialis	Musculocutaneous	(C4)C5,6(C7)	None
Biceps brachii	Musculocutaneous	(C4)C5,6(C7)	Flexion of the supinated forearm against resistance
Triceps	Radial	(C5)C6-C8	Resistance to extension of elbows from varying positions of flexion

*Numbers in parentheses indicate a variable but not rare contribution.

peripheral nerve function, sensory evaluation, and testing of reflex arcs (Table 5-1). Evaluation of the sympathetic chain may reveal findings suggestive of dystrophy. The extent of the neurological examination depends upon the clinical presentation.

Muscle Testing

To localize a lesion, a detailed knowledge of the anatomy and variations of the brachial plexus and its contributing cervical and thoracic roots is necessary to evaluate fully muscle deficits following injury or disease. In a patient with a brachial plexus injury, this examination is very detailed. By contrast, the patient with degenerative cervical disease with encroachment on one nerve root will have characteristic findings to localize the lesion (Table 5-2). Extensive tables are available to assist in determining the problem when required (Tables 5-1 to 5-3).

Sensory Testing

The loss of skin sensation may be due either to peripheral nerve damage or encroachment on cervical nerve roots. The pattern of peripheral nerve cutaneous innervation is well-documented and denervation has an easily definable area. In contrast, selective cervical root involvement is less easily defined due to dermatomal overlap. Dermatomal maps have been formulated either by sectioning nerves above and below the segmental level (Foerster's charts), or by selective division of cervical nerve roots and observation of the area of altered sensation (Keegan's map) (Fig. 5-11). A simplified pattern of dermatomes for the upper extremities is: C5, lateral deltoid; C6, thumb; C7, middle finger; C8, little finger; and T1, inner aspect proximal arm.

Reflexes

Several reflexes in the upper extremities are available for testing the integrity of neural arcs. Some are specific such as the biceps jerk, whereas others are testing gross motion responses (e.g., the clavicular reflex). The quality of the reflex should also be noted: is it brisk as might occur in thyrotoxicosis, or is it sluggish as in myxedema?

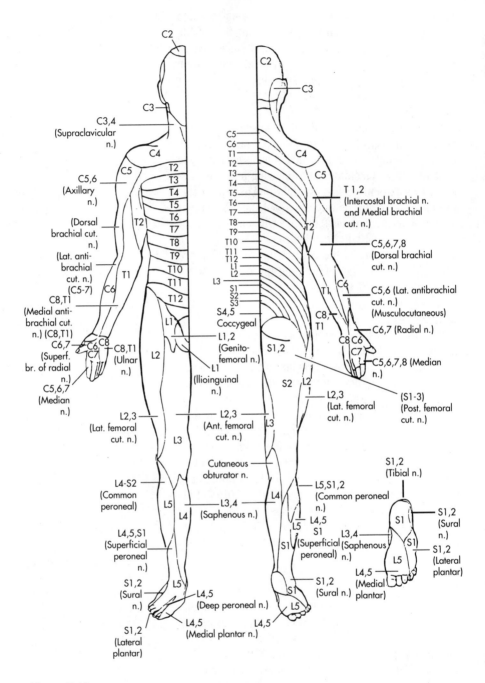

Figure 5-11.
Cutaneous dermatomes.

Biceps Reflex

The patient's arm is flexed at the elbow. The examiner's thumb is over the biceps tendon insertion and this is tapped with the hammer. The biceps muscle normally contracts **(Fig. 5-7)**. The neurological cervical root level is C5, but mostly C6. The peripheral nerve is the musculocutaneous.

Triceps Reflex

The patient's arm is supported with the elbow flexed to 90 degrees. The triceps insertion is struck with a hammer and an extensor response evoked **(Fig. 5-12)**. The cervical roots are C6-C8 with predominant representation of C7. The peripheral nerve is the radial.

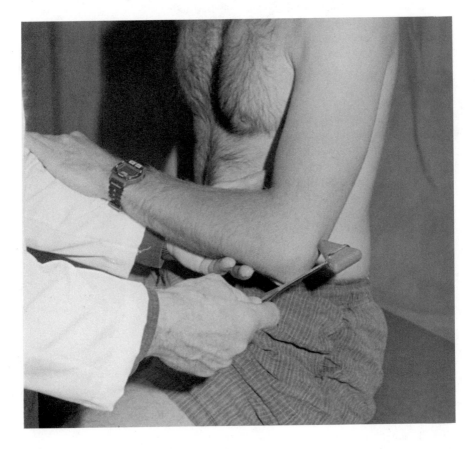

Figure 5-12.
The triceps reflex is elicited by the examiner cradling the patient's arm and then striking over the triceps insertion.

Brachioradialis Reflex

With the forearm relaxed in a neutral position, the tendon of the brachioradialis is struck approximately 2 to 3 cm proximal to the radial styloid. In response to this is the contraction with associated elbow flexion or wrist radial deviation. Its peripheral innervation is from the radial nerve and C5-C6 root components.

Pectoralis Reflex

The patient's arm is abducted 20 to 30 degrees and supported by the examiner. The physician's thumb is placed over the distal tendon of the pectoralis major muscle and the thumb is tapped with the hammer. Contraction of the muscle is seen and felt, which causes the arm to adduct and to slightly internally rotate. The pectoralis major is innervated by both medial and lateral pectoral nerves and has myotomes from C5-C7 supplying the clavicular and manubrial portions and C8-T1 supplies the lower sternal portions.

Scapular Reflex

The patient stands with the arm abducted 15 to 20 degrees. The inferior angle of the scapula is tapped, the scapula moves medially, and the arm adducts due to the action of the rhomboids plus other muscles. In a very muscular individual, this test may be difficult to interpret and a negative response may be insignificant.

Clavicular Reflex

Tapping the lateral portion of the clavicle may result in contraction of various muscles in the arm. It can be used for demonstrating differences in irritability of deep reflexes between the two upper limbs.

Moro Reflex

This reflex is useful in evaluating gross motor responses in an infant (**Fig. 5-10**). The reflex is present at birth but disappears in 10 to 20 weeks. The infant is laid supine and the head supported in the slightly flexed position. The head is dropped quickly but gently into slight extension; in response to this, the upper limbs show slight abduction, extension, and circumduction with flexion of the lower limb, that is, a startled response. If a brachial plexus lesion, fractured clavicle, or hemiparesis of a limb is present, this reflex will be absent or asymmetrical.

Horner's Syndrome

Injury or disease at the base of the neck may cause damage to the cervical sympathetic chain at the sixth cervical level. Here is found an ipsilateral dilatation (myosis) of the pupil with ptosis of the upper eyelid and lack of facial sweating (anhydrosis) **(Fig. 5-13)**.

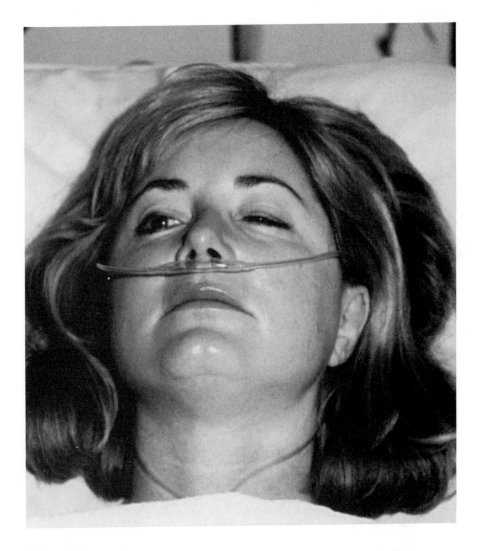

Figure 5-13.
Horner's syndrome consists of ipsilateral dilation (myosis) of the pupil with ptosis of the upper eyelid and lack of facial sweating (anhydrosis).

TABLE 5-4
PERIPHERAL NERVE ASSESSMENT
OF UPPER EXTREMITIES

Nerve	Muscle Tested	Test	Sensory Innervation
Axillary	Deltoid	Resisted shoulder abduction	Lateral aspect upper arm
Radial	Metacarpophalangeal extensors	Resisted extension metacarpophalangeal joints	Dorsal web space of thumb
Median	Thenar muscles	Resisted palmar abduction of thumb	Palmar tip of index finger
Ulnar	First dorsal interosseous	Resisted adduction index finger	Ulnar aspect distal baby finger

Peripheral Nerve Assessment of Upper Extremities

To assess peripheral nerve problems in the upper extremities, muscles and motions can be tested. To assess strength, muscles that are most commonly innervated by a particular peripheral nerve can be isolated and reliably tested (Tables 5-2 to 5-4).

Sometimes in musculoskeletal problems the hand is wrapped and immobilized, and only the thumb is available for testing. In such circumstances the principles of the RUM thumb can be applied neurologically to assess radial, ulnar, and median nerves. For the radial nerve, it is extension of the DIP joint of the thumb, for the ulnar nerve, adduction of the thumb or assessment of Froment's paper sign (Fig. 5-14, A, B) and for the median nerve, flexion of the DIP joint.

Thoracic Levels

In traumatic injuries to the thoracic spine or in malignant conditions in this area, the examiner must understand the sensory levels of thoracic involvement, which are illustrated on the dermatomes involved in the thoracic spine in Fig. 5-11.

Text continued on p. 168.

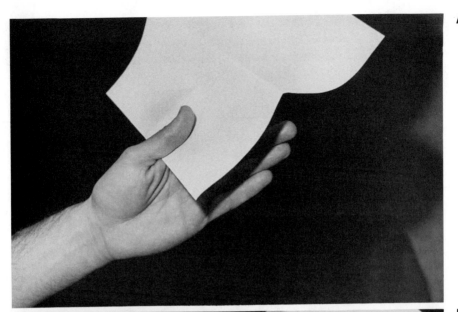

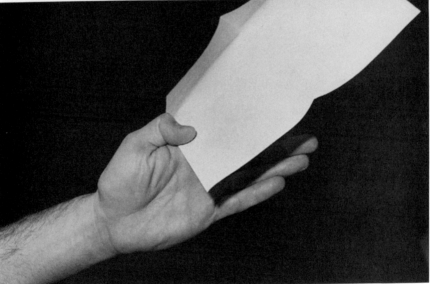

Figure 5-14.

A,B, Froment's paper sign is determined by asking the patient to hold a piece of paper between thumb and interosseous area or index finger. The patient with a normal functioning ulnar nerve keeps the thumb straight, as demonstrated in A, whereas the patient with a deficient ulnar nerve flexes the distal interphalangeal (DIP) joint to capture the piece of paper, as illustrated in B.

TABLE 5-5
MUSCLE TESTING CHART FOR LOWER EXTREMITIES

Muscle	Innervation (Peripheral Nerve)	Myotomes (Roots)	Technique for Testing
Psoas major	Lumbar plexus	L1-L4	With thigh flexed, raise knee against resistance
Iliacus	Femoral	L2-L4	With patient supine, raise extended extremity against downward resistance upon thigh
Quadriceps femoris	Femoral	L2-L4	Sitting or supine, extend leg against downward resistance against leg
Sartorius	Femoral	L2-L4	With knee extended, resist hip flexion*
Rectus femoris	Femoral	L2-L4	Resist extended leg
Gluteus maximus	Inferior gluteal	L5-S1	Resist hip extension with patient prone
Gluteus medius	Superior gluteal	L4-S1	Resist hip abduction; sitting or supine separate knees against resistance
Gluteus minimus	Superior gluteal	L4-S1	Resist hip abduction
Tensor fascia latae	Superior gluteal	C4-S1	Resist hip abduction
Piriformis	To piriformis	S1-S2	Resist lateral rotation, abduction of hip

*Muscles act in groups and often may be tested in groups.

TABLE 5-5
MUSCLE TESTING CHART
FOR LOWER EXTREMITIES – cont'd.

Muscle	Innervation (Peripheral Nerve)	Myotomes (Roots)	Technique for Testing
Adductor longus	Obturator	L2-L4	Sitting or supine with knees together, patient resists separation of knees
Adductor brevis	Obturator	L2-L4	Same test as noted above
Adductor magnus	Obturator	L2-L4	Resist adduction and extension of hip
Gracilis	Obturator	L2-L4	Resist thigh adduction
Gastrocnemius	Tibial	L5-S2	Patient extends knee while plantar flexing foot against resistance; palpate muscle while testing
Soleus	Tibial	L5-S2	Resist plantar foot flexion (same as above)
Biceps femoris	Tibial	L5-S1	While sitting, flex knee against resistance or while prone with knee partly flexed, further flex against resistance
Semitendinosus	Tibial	L5-S1	With hip extended, resist knee flexion and medial rotation
Semimembranosus	Tibial	L5-S1	Same test as noted above
Tibialis anterior	Deep peroneal	L4-S1	Dorsiflex and invert foot against resistance

Continued.

TABLE 5-5
MUSCLE TESTING CHART
FOR LOWER EXTREMITIES – cont'd.

Muscle	Innervation (Peripheral Nerve)	Myotomes (Roots)	Technique for Testing
Peroneus tertius	Deep peroneal	L4-S1	With foot dorsiflexed, resist eversion
Extensor digitorum longus	Deep peroneal	L4-S1	Resist toe extension
Extensor hallucis longus	Deep peroneal	L4-S1	Resist big toe extension
Extensor digitorum brevis	Deep peroneal	L4-S1	Resist toe extension
Extensor hallucis brevis	Deep peroneal	L4-S1	Resist big toe extension
Peroneus longus	Superficial peroneal	L4-S1	With foot in plantar flexion resist eversion
Peroneus brevis	Superficial peroneal	L4-S1	Same test as above
Tibialis posterior	Posterior tibial	L5-S1	While foot is plantar flexed, resist inversion
Flexor digitorum longus	Posterior tibial	L5-S1	Resist plantar flexion of toes
Flexor hallucis longus	Posterior tibial	L5-S2	Resist plantar flexion of big toe

TABLE 5-6
NEUROLOGICAL ROOT LEVELS
IN THE LOWER EXTREMITIES

Level	Motor	Sensory	Reflex
L2	Hip adductors	Anterior groin	None
L3	Hip flexors	Anterior thigh	Knee
L4	Ankle dorsiflexion	Medial border lower limb	None
L5	Toe extension	Web space and second toe, lateral border of foot	None
S1	Ankle plantar flexion	Sole of foot	Ankle

TABLE 5-7
PERIPHERAL NERVE ASSESSMENT
OF LOWER EXTREMITIES

Nerve	Muscle Tested	Test	Sensory Innervation
Obturator nerve	Hip adductors	Resisted adduction hip	Anterior groin
Femoral nerve	Knee extension	Resisted knee extension	Anterior thigh
Posterior tibial nerve	Ankle plantar flexion	Resisted ankle plantar flexion	—
Anterior tibial nerve	Ankle dorsiflexion	Resisted ankle dorsiflexion	Dorsal aspect big toe web space
Peroneal nerve	Ankle eversion	Resisted ankle eversion	Lateral border distal foot

Neurological Examination of Lower Limbs

Assessment of neurological function of the lower limbs involves motor, sensory, and reflex determinations (Tables 5-5 to 5-7). Manifestations of neurological involvement of the lower limbs may reveal either upper or lower motor neuron problems. For example, the patient with atlantoaxial instability secondary to rheumatoid arthritis may reveal increased spasticity in the legs manifest as increased tone, heightened reflexes (Fig. 5-1), sustained clonus (Fig. 5-2), or upgoing toes (Fig. 5-3). Bowel and bladder involvement is critical and suggests a very careful neurological assessment. Loss of rectal tone may be present with a cauda equina lesion or loss of the bulbocavernosus reflex may follow a thoracolumbar fracture dislocation.

The method of muscle testing, sensory examination, and reflex assessment are comparable to those described in the upper extremity. The tables included will clarify those issues.

Peripheral Nerve Testing

Similar to the upper extremities, peripheral nerve testing of the lower extremities is important and is included in the testing of muscles of the lower extremity controlling motion (Table 5-7).

Chapter

6   Stability (Laxity) Assessment

The stability or instability of a joint, depending upon the underlying pathology, may be a major consideration when examining the musculoskeletal system. This is applicable to an anterior cruciate ligament tear in the knee with resulting giving way. Stability assessment would not be very important in osteoarthritis of the hip, yet newborns require a specialized approach to stability assessment of the hip. A spectrum of stability exists from stiffness to generalized joint laxity, resulting in a continuum of normal joint translation or laxity to clinical subluxation or frank dislocation. The examiner should bear in mind, however, that laxity or translation, even if significant, does not necessarily imply instability. An appreciation of what is normal and abnormal allows the application of specific methods that stress or load joints, thereby allowing the physician to determine their clinical significance. Excessive motion at a point such as 20 degrees of recurvatum of the knee may suggest loose jointedness. Perhaps the best indication of deficient collagen tissue that may relate to instability is an ability to abduct the thumb to the forearm **(Fig. 6-1)**. A measurement of less than 4 cm indicates increased flexibility. Clinical instability or laxity and translation on physical examination may be manifest in various clinical instability tests, including angular stress testing, translation testing, apprehension testing, and patient demonstration.

Clinical Instability Tests
Angular Stress Testing
Angular stress can be determined by applying angular stress to the joint and stressing the joint beyond the normal confines of that ligament and feeling or visually observing the abnormal angular movement. This occurs

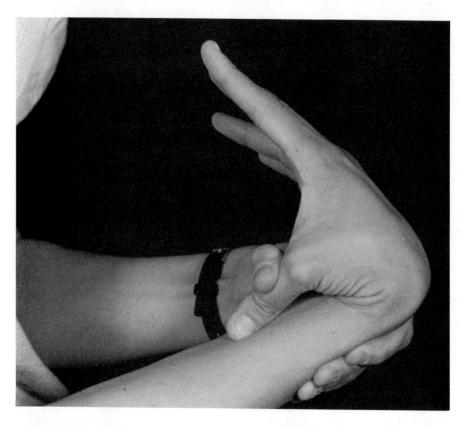

Figure 6-1.
This demonstrates an ability to have the thumb passively touch the forearm, suggestive of ligamentous instability or excessive flexibility of a part. This is probably the best test to assess excessive joint flexibility.

with medial instability of the knee, demonstrated by a valgus stress (**Fig. 6-2, A, B**) or ulnar collateral ligament instability of the thumb (**Fig. 6-3**). When applying angular stress, the physician may note either an increase in angle compared with the opposite extremity or in increase of millimeters of opening in the joint surfaces. For example, with a valgus stress applied to the knee, the space between the medial femoral condyle and the medial tibial plateau is measured. Classically in the knee, medial opening has been accepted as

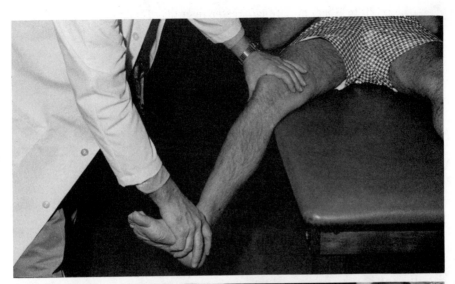

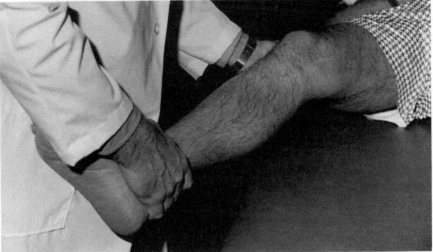

Figure 6-2.
A, This illustrates the determination of medial collateral ligament instability of the knee by applying an angular stress with the leg resting on the top of the examining table. B, This demonstrates medial collateral ligament insufficiency by applying an angular stress, estimating the millimeters of opening medially. Counterpressure is applied with the left hand against the outside of the knee and stress applied with the right hand in a handshaking relationship with the ankle. This test is performed at 0 and 30 degrees of flexion.

- Grade I, 0 to 5 mm of opening greater than the opposite side
- Grade II, 5 to 10 mm of opening greater than the opposite side
- Grade III, greater than 10 mm of opening when compared to the opposite side, the last situation suggesting a complete medial disruption if an acute injury

Recently, the International Knee Documentation Study (IKDS) has instituted a slightly modified grading system, based on both instrumented and manual testing. The IKDS has four grades:

- Grade 0, 0 to 2 mm greater than the normal side, D, or difference
- Grade I, 3 to 5 mm greater than the normal side
- Grade II, 6 to 10 mm greater than the normal side
- Grade III, 10 mm greater than the normal side

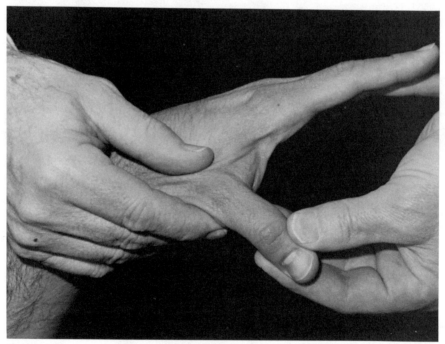

Figure 6-3.
Deficiency of the ulnar collateral ligament is demonstrated by applying an angular stress.

Estimating the opening of each knee in millimeters and indicating which is abnormal with the sign D and indicating that the grading is based on this difference may be helpful.

In addition to this objective measurement or feel with stressing, the physician must also appreciate whether the end point is soft or firm. This feel is more useful immediately following an acute injury and, if a soft end point, suggests a complete disruption.

Translation Testing

The examiner may be able to sublux, dislocate, or excessively translate a joint indicating abnormal trans-

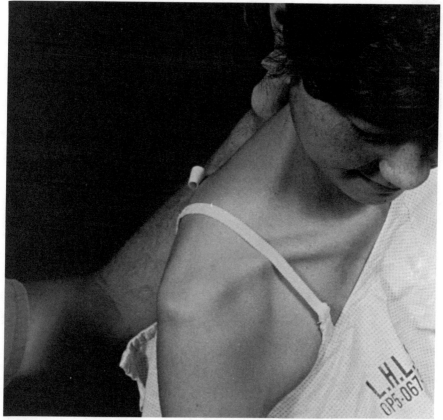

Figure 6-4.
Translation is the movement of a part parallel to a fixed point on the opposite part. This patient demonstrates excessive inferior translation of the humeral head in the glenoid fossa, suggestive of multidirectional instability.

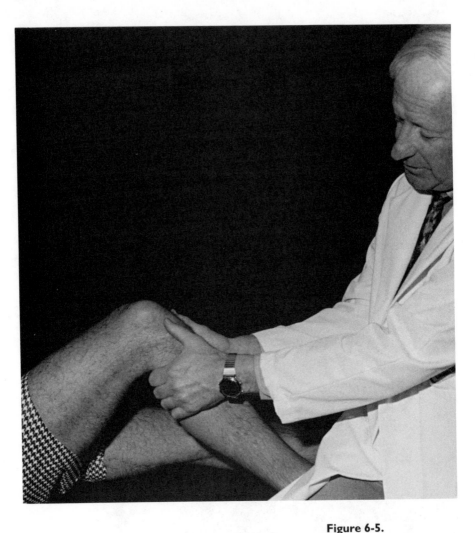

Figure 6-5.
An anterior drawer sign demonstrates excessive anterior translation of the tibial plateau relative to the femur.

lation of the part or actual instability. Translation is the movement of a part parallel to a fixed point on the opposite part (i.e., one side of a joint moving parallel relative to the opposite side of a joint). This may be demonstrated with significant inferior translation of the humeral head in the glenoid in the patient with multidirectional instability **(Fig. 6-4)**. It may also be demonstrated in a newborn who has an unstable hip, allowing it to be subluxed, dislocated, and often relocated. Anterior drawer of the knee with an anterior

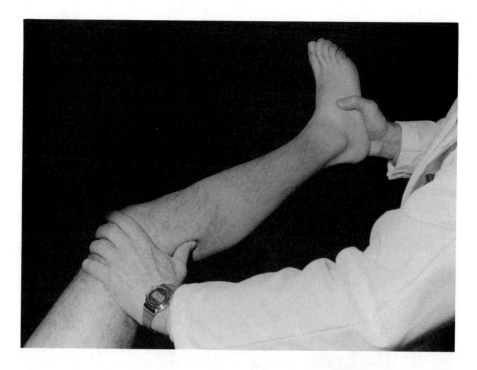

Figure 6-6.
Once a special test, pivot shift maneuvers have become a routine part of stability assessment of the knee.

cruciate ligament deficiency is another example of translating the joint beyond normal **(Fig. 6-5)**. Translation might be the term to describe this testing with subluxation and dislocation reserved for the clinical diagnosis of instability. In a person who actively participates in sports, the knee requires particular attention to stability assessment consisting of most of the described techniques. The pivot shift maneuver has now become a routine part of stability assessment of the knee, rather than a special test **(Fig. 6-6)**.

Apprehension Testing

Stressing the joint or part so that it is about to dislocate or sublux may produce the sensation of impending subluxation or dislocation or what is known as an apprehension sign. This is applicable to patellar instability of the knee **(Fig. 6-7)** or recurrent anterior instability of the shoulder **(Fig. 6-8, A, B, C)**. Although pain may occur with such testing, it should not be confused with or interpreted as apprehension.

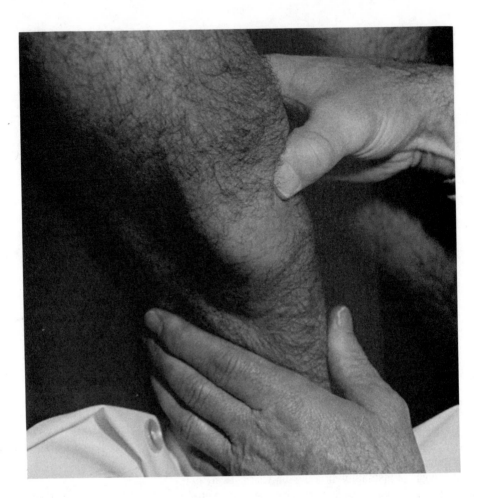

Figure 6-7.
By applying a lateral stress to the patella, the physician can sometimes elicit apprehension on the part of the patient, which is suggestive of underlying patellar instability.

Figure 6-8.
A, The apprehension or crank test is performed by having the fingers over the humeral head and the thumb levering or pushing the humeral head from behind and the examiner forcibly externally rotating in the abducted position. A feeling of apprehension, that something very worrisome is about to happen, suggests anterior instability. B, C, The fulcrum test, also an apprehension test, can be performed supine with the patient's body as a counterweight, the table edge as the fulcrum, and the arm as the lever. With progressive external rotation in the abducted position, the patient may have an apprehensive reaction or a feeling that an instability episode is about to occur.

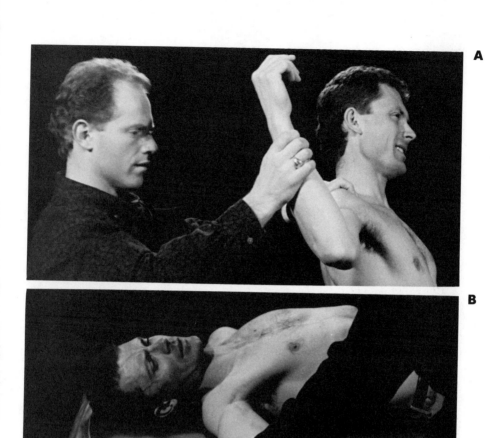

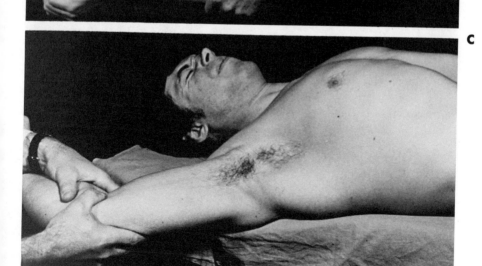

Figure 6-8.

Patient Demonstration

The patient, by postural positioning, may be able to demonstrate instability of a part. The patient with posterior shoulder instability can frequently demonstrate the instability by arm position or muscular contraction (Fig. 6-9, A, B). Similarly, patients who have posterolateral instability of the knee and a dramatically positive reverse pivot shift can frequently demonstrate that instability by fixing the foot to the floor with the knee flexed 90 degrees and then pivoting the tibial plateau (Fig. 6-10).

At this point, examples of stability assessment of each of the important joints, commencing with the shoulder, may prove helpful. *Laxity* and *translation* imply similar movements; they vary greatly among patients and do not in themselves define instability. They are biomechanical terms. *Instability* is a clinical term based on the patient's complaints and supplemented with the presence of some of these signs.

A
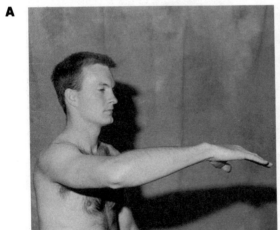

B
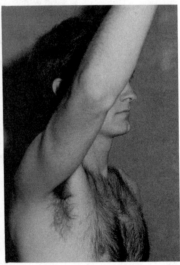

Figure 6-9.
A, The patient with posterior shoulder instability can often demonstrate this instability by forward flexing the arm in the internally rotated position. In this position, the humeral head is subluxed posteriorly. B, Continuing toward the coronal plane of the body elicits a clunk, which is a reduction of this posteriorly subluxed shoulder.

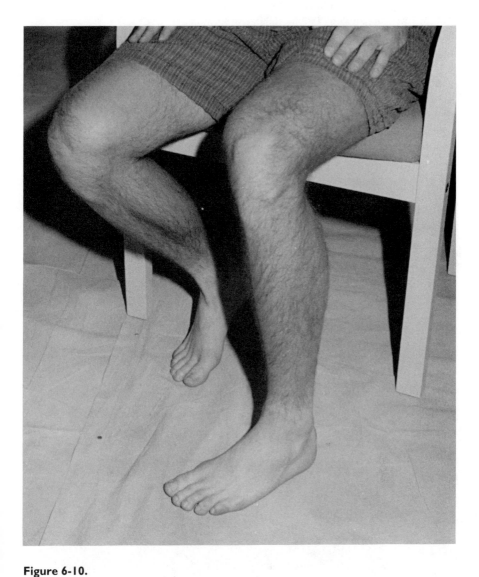

Figure 6-10.
Patients who have posterolateral instability can sometimes demonstrate a reverse pivot shift phenomena with the knee flexed and their foot on the floor. Rarely, patients with anterior cruciate deficiency can demonstrate such a phenomena, which would actually be a pivot shift.

Stability Assessment of the Shoulder

The assessment of stability of the glenohumeral joint requires consideration by two methods. The first is to document the amount of passive translation of the humeral head in the glenoid fossa when stressed by the examiner. The global mobility of the shoulder can allow laxity of the shoulder to occur in at least three possible directions: anterior, posterior, or inferior; the last is often associated with multidirectional laxity. Any reproduction of symptoms appreciated by the patient

A

B

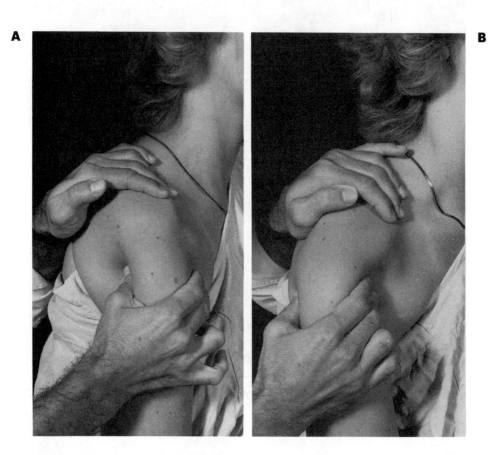

Figure 6-11.

A, B, Anterior and posterior translation of the glenohumeral joint can be determined with the load and shift test. A demonstrates anterior translation or anterior drawer testing of the humeral head in the fossa, while B demonstrates posterior translation of the humeral head in the glenoid fossa.

with those maneuvers is significant. The second is to attempt production of apprehension by stressing the shoulder in provocative positions of compromise.

Glenohumeral Translation (Load and Shift Test)

Glenohumeral translation should be examined in both the upright **(Fig. 6-11, A, B)** and supine **(Fig. 6-12)** positions. The mobility of the scapula on the thoracic wall and gross movement of the entire shoulder girdle with stressing can make assessment of such translation difficult. Although the scapula can be fixed to some degree to provide an appreciation of translation, it should not be rigidly fixed. This is comparable to the pivot shift maneuver in the knee, where both tibia and femur must have some independence of movement for an accurate assessment of the pivot shift. With practice, the clinician will develop an appreciation and feel for glenohumeral translation.

When assessing the amount of translation, the humeral head must be initially reduced concentrically into the glenoid fossa (i.e., "loaded"). In patients with scarring from previous surgery, the humeral head may have a resting position that is not concentric but sitting anterior, posterior, and inferior. Likewise, the very lax individual, while supine and under anesthesia, may

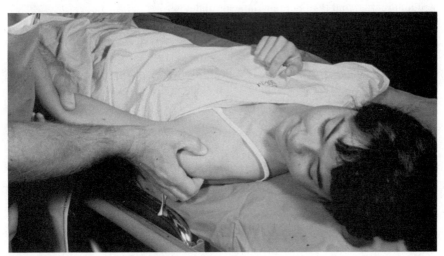

Figure 6-12.
Glenohumeral translation can be performed in the supine position.

have the humeral head rest posterior to the glenoid fossa. Hence, at the start of any stress testing, the humeral head must be secured and pushed into the glenoid fossa to ensure its reduction to the neutral position. Once the humeral head is loaded, directional stress may be applied. As either anterior or posterior stress is increased, the head may be felt to ride up to and sometimes over the glenoid rim (Fig. 6-11, A, B). This may be difficult to appreciate because an associated movement of the shoulder girdle is usually present. Similarly, as in all other joints, muscular or obese individuals may prove difficult to assess. For recording and describing this translation, some form of grading system is helpful.

The technique for this part of the examination initially involves assessment with the patient sitting and the examiner located just beside and behind the side to be examined. The normal or asymptomatic shoulder should be examined first to provide a baseline and to demonstrate the maneuver to the patient to allay possible anxieties. The examiner's hand is placed over the shoulder and scapula to steady the limb girdle; with the opposite hand, the examiner then grasps the humeral head between the thumb and fingers (Fig. 6-13). The head is "loaded" by applied pressure in a medial direction and then both an anterior and posterior translational stress is applied noting the amount of translation. Next, the elbow is grasped and inferior traction is applied. The area adjacent to the acromion is observed and dimpling of the skin may indicate a sulcus sign (Fig. 6-14, A, B). The acromion and the humeral head underneath are palpated to gain an impression, in centimeters, of the amount of inferior humeral translation.

Glenohumeral translation is also assessed with the patient supine (Fig. 6-12). Here the arm is grasped and positioned in approximately 20 degrees abduction 20 degrees of forward flexion in neutral rotation. The humeral head is loaded, then posterior and anterior stresses applied. Translation must be assessed with the arm in different positions, for example, in external rotation and abduction. Excess translation in this position compared with the opposite side may be more meaningful than in the neutral position. Similarly, in the supine position, inferior stress is applied, again noting the sulcus sign. The accuracy of these tests depends both on the examiner's skill and the patient's ability to relax. In some patients with associated tendinitis, grasping the humeral head between the thumb and fingers is too painful. In these situations, grasping the upper arm distal to the shoulder may be the only method of assessing translation, but it is less reliable.

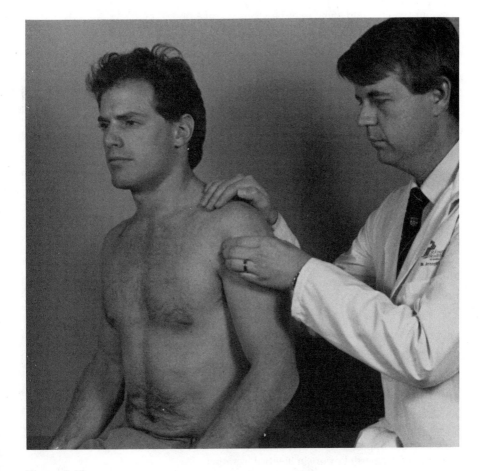

Figure 6-13.
The load and shift test is performed sitting with the shoulder girdle stabilized with one hand on top of the shoulder over the clavicle and scapula and the opposite hand grasping the humeral head between thumb and index finger. A stress is then applied following loading of the head into the fossa.

Documentation of Anterioposterior Translation

Using a clinical grading system of translation is helpful. Using distance or percentages, unless determined radiographically (and radiographic determination in such patients is impractical) is not practical and is too subjective. Two important clinical happenings occur: (1) the examiner feels the humeral head ride up the face to the glenoid rim (Grade I), and (2), the head can actually be felt riding over the glenoid rim but reduces with release of the stress (Grade II). A small amount of translation should not be given a grade or could be noted as Grade 0. If the humeral head remains

A 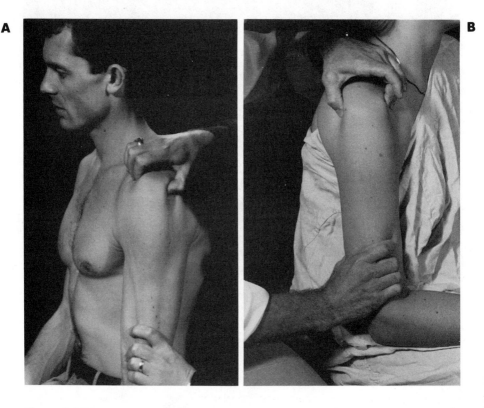 **B**

Figure 6-14.
A, B, The sulcus sign is assessed by the examiner applying longitudinal traction to the upper arm and noting the distance the humeral head moves away from the acromion. Both shoulders reveal approximately 2 cm of inferior translation.

out of this joint when stress is released, this should be noted, but for simplicity not given a separate grade. Patients with multidirectional instability usually have Grade II translation, although some normal patients can have Grade II. Having determined the degree of glenohumeral joint translation, these findings must be correlated with the patient's symptoms.

Documentation of Inferior Translation of the Sulcus Sign

Because the joint is not loaded, appreciating the humeral head riding up the face of the glenoid or over the rim with inferior stress is more difficult. Clinically, estimating the distance the upper part of the humeral head moves away from the undersurface of the acromion is crude but more reliable. The physician can force the thumb and finger in between the acromion and humeral head to further depress the humeral head and appreciate whether it moves less than 1 cm (Grade 0), more than 1 cm (Grade I), or more than 2 cm (Grade II). This then requires documentation (Fig. 6-14, A, B).

In the relaxed or anesthetized patient, most normal shoulders will allow some translation of the humeral head in the glenoid fossa. Many shoulders can be translated posteriorly up to half the width of the glenoid fossa (i.e., the examiner can feel the humeral head ride up the glenoid face and sometimes even over the glenoid rim). The physician should apply a grading system and, under anesthesia, normal shoulders would have mild translation anteriorly and inferiorly and up to moderate posteriorly. Even normal shoulders may have what seems to be excessive translation in all three directions. In most patients, especially if they are relaxed, a good correlation of translation awake and under anesthesia exists, especially inferior and posterior. Accurate determination in the painful shoulder may only be possible under anesthesia.

Apprehension Tests and Symptomatic Translation

In addition to assessing stability by reproducing the symptom complex with translation, the examiner should also attempt to elicit apprehension with stressing in certain provocative positions of impending subluxation or dislocation.

The most common direction of instability is anterior. The usual position of the arm when subluxation or dislocation occurs is abduction and external rotation. The apprehension test for anterior instability can be performed both in the upright (**Fig. 6-8, A**) and supine (**Fig. 6-8, B, C**) positions, although maximal muscle relaxation is best achieved with the patient supine. With the patient sitting, the examiner stands or sits behind the shoulder to be examined. To assess the patient's left shoulder, the examiner raises the arm to 90 degrees of abduction and begins to rotate the humerus externally. The examiner's right hand is placed over the humeral head with the thumb pushing from posterior for extra leverage, however, with the fingers anterior to control any sudden instability episode that may occur. With increasing external rotation and controlled gentle forward pressure exerted against the humeral head, an impending feeling of anterior instability may be produced (i.e., an apprehension sign). This may be referred to as the crank test (**Fig. 6-8, A**). An apprehensive look may appear on the patient's face or he may contract his muscles to prevent dislocation, or he may fear that if the stress is continued the shoulder will "come out." Pain alone is not a positive apprehension sign, although it is often present.

This test can be repeated with the patient supine (referred to as a fulcrum test). The shoulder to be examined is positioned so that the scapula is supported by the edge of the examining table and the proximal humerus is then stressed in varying degrees of abduction and external rotation, attempting to reproduce impending instability. In the supine position (**Fig. 6-8, B, C**), the body acts as the counterweight; the edge of the table, the fulcrum; and the arm, the lever. When the apprehensive position is located, note is taken of the amount of external rotation. With the arm in this position, a posterior stress may be exerted on the proximal humerus and the apprehension may disappear allowing more external humeral rotation before reemergence of the apprehension sign (**Fig. 6-15, A, B**). This Fowler's sign, or relocation test, has two possible explanations: at the apprehension point the humeral head is slightly subluxed and pushing it posteriorly causes reduction, or the posteriorly directed pressure acts as a supportive buttress anteriorly to

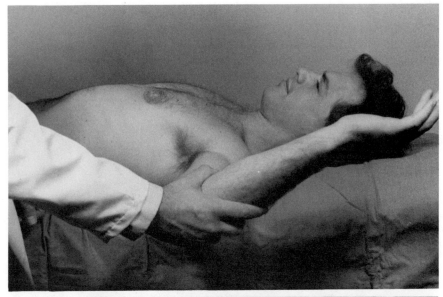

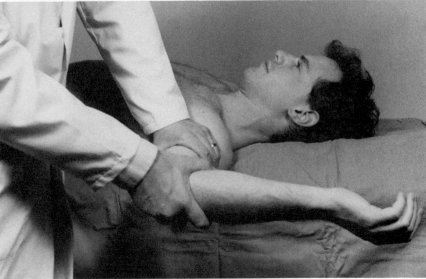

Figure 6-15.
A, The relocation test is documented by stressing the arm in external rotation and abduction, looking for a reaction of pain. B, By then pushing posteriorly on the proximal humerus, the physician either relocates the humeral head or butresses the humeral head, allowing more external rotation in this position with less pain. This positive relocation test might also be applied to the apprehension sign.

give the patient more confidence, lessening the pain and/or apprehension. These apprehension signs are most commonly applied to patients with anterior shoulder instability. In the throwing athlete, some examiners believe that if pain, even in the absence of apprehension, is produced with this stressing, anterior subluxation is a possible diagnosis. A positive relocation test allows greater external rotation in abduction with less pain and further suggests anterior subluxation. If the posteriorly pushed upper arm is suddenly released when stressed in external rotation and abduction, the patient may have a dramatic increase in the pain, termed a *release test,* which may be caused by the humeral head jumping forward upon release of the posteriorly applied stress. Similarly, the pain can be augmented with external rotation and abduction by pulling forward on the back of the arm, termed *augmentation test.* These findings do not represent the classical apprehension sign, which is fairly accurate for anterior instability. With pain alone, its meaning, along with relocation, augmentation, and release testing are much less reliable for anterior instability.

Posterior instability is a subluxation rather than a dislocation and if recurrent can usually be demonstrated by the patient, either by arm positioning in forward elevation or by selective muscular control in various positions of elevation and internal rotation. Having ascertained the compromising maneuver, the examiner may attempt to reproduce the instability by manually duplicating the stresses **(Fig. 6-16)**. Apprehension is uncommon in this position. In patients with posterior instability, posterior translation is usually up to and over the rim and almost always reproduces the symptoms of the patient. It is surprising, however, how in some patients, translation does not go over the rim and yet the patient still appreciates that as the direction of the instability. Because this is usually a painless subluxation that easily reduces, apprehension is not commonly present and therefore not a reliable sign. With posterior stress, patients who are in pain may resist, and this is sometimes erroneously interpreted as apprehension. In posterior instability, the patient who cannot demonstrate the instability may present a diagnostic challenge. In these patients, posterior translation of the humeral head on the glenoid with repro-

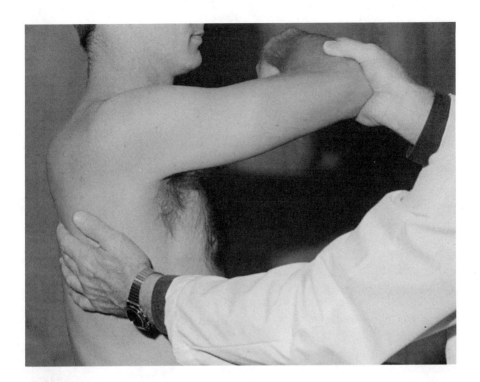

Figure 6-16.
In the presence of posterior subluxation, the examiner can sometimes duplicate this maneuver by elevating the arm and pushing posteriorly. Moving the arm toward the coronal plane reduces the posterior subluxation. With this testing, posterior apprehension is uncommon.

duction of the symptom complex of the humeral head, "coming out" may provide the only clue to the diagnosis (**Fig. 6-11, B**). Patients with added inferior instability may say that distal traction on the arm reproduces their symptom complex suggesting underlying additional multidirectional instability (**Fig. 6-14, B**).

Stability Assessment of the Knee

The knee is perhaps the most common joint to be examined for stability. As in the shoulder, an organized format to assess knee stability is important. The segments of the stability assessment of the knee into its various components actually starts with range of motion already performed. For example, the presence of hyperextension or recurvatum, particularly greater on one side when compared to a normal side, may be suggestive of ligamentous instability **(Fig. 6-17)**. The specific components of the examination may be divided into sections. Whether the patient is awake or under anesthesia, the following outline can be followed in an organized approach when examining a knee for instability.

A. With a relatively straight or slightly flexed knee, the physician examines for
    1. Valgus and varus in 0 degrees **(Fig. 6-2, B)**
    2. Valgus and varus at 30 degrees of flexion **(Figs. 6-2, B, 6-18, A, B)**
    3. Lachman in 20 to 30 degrees of flexion **(Fig. 6-19)**

B. Translation and rotational testing at 90 degrees of flexion, consists of
    1. Anterior drawer **(Fig. 6-5)**

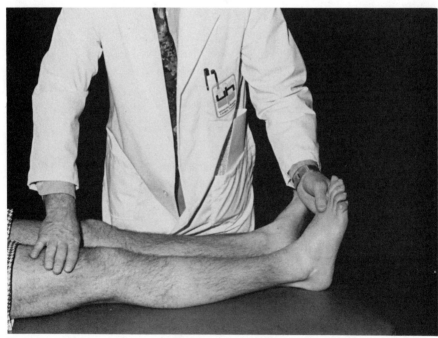

Figure 6-17.
Hyperextension or recurvatum of the knee passively greater on one side may be suggestive of ligamentous laxity.

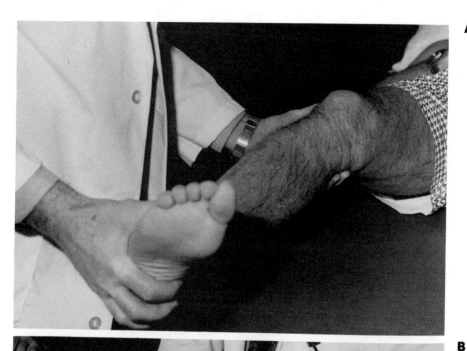

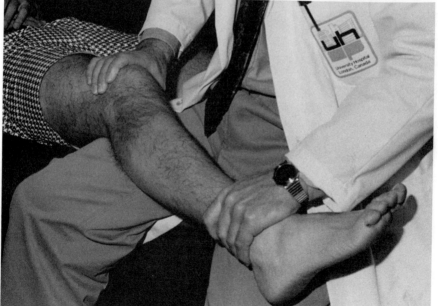

Figure 6-18.
A, B, These positions demonstrate two methods of eliciting
varus instability with lateral ligamentous disruption both at
30 degrees of flexion.

2. Posterior drawer
3. Anterior and posterior drawering in external and internal rotation

C. Pivot shift maneuvers such as
   1. MacIntosh (Fig. 6-20)
   2. Losee maneuver (Fig. 6-21)
   3. Flexion/rotation (Fig. 6-22)
   4. Other pivot shift tests

D. Specialized testing for ligamentous instability
   1. Posterolateral instability testing (Fig. 6-23, A, B, C)
   2. Reverse pivot testing (Fig. 6-24)
   3. Dynamic anterior cruciate testing (Fig. 6-25, A, B)
   4. Quadriceps active or dynamic resistance testing for posterior cruciate (Fig. 6-26)

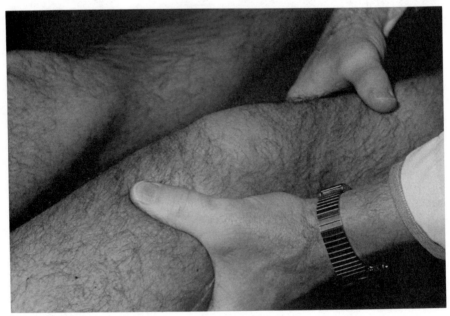

Figure 6-19.
This demonstrates the Lachman test performed by pulling forward on the tibia with the knee at approximately 20 to 30 degrees of flexion. If positive, this is indicative of anterior cruciate insufficiency.

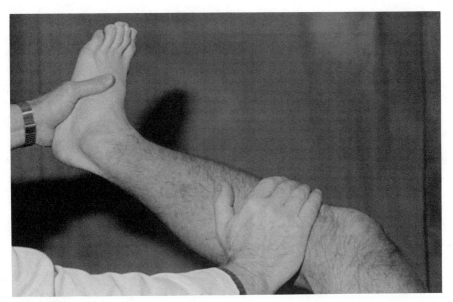

Figure 6-20.
The MacIntosh or original pivot shift maneuver is a reduction phenomenon, wherein the leg is taken from full extension to a flexed position. At approximately 30 degrees, the tibial plateau reduces.

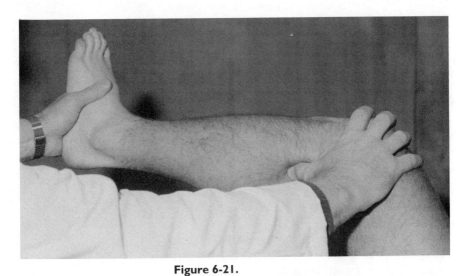

Figure 6-21.
The Losee maneuver is a subluxation phenomenon where the leg is taken from the flexed to the extended position. The tibia subluxes at about 30 degrees of flexion with a valgus axial load.

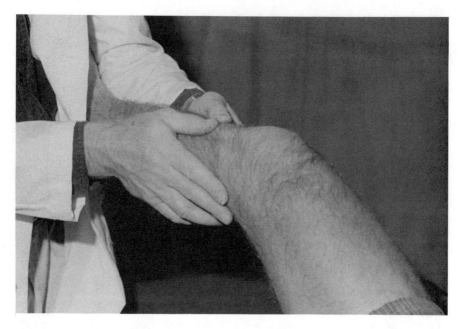

Figure 6-22.
The two-part flexion rotation test consists of a reverse Lachman test and a pivoting phenomenon with the application of valgus and axial loading.

Both knees must be examined for comparative purposes because assessment of ligamentous instability rating and grading historically has been based on the opposite normal extremity. This is particularly so with the exception of pivot shift maneuvers, which are graded in isolation on each side. The recent IKDS suggests a grading system as previously described, whether instrumented or manual in four different grades. The new proposed system considers delta or difference, D, to indicate the abnormal knee in describing the findings in both knees so that the reader can better compare.

Initially, the knee should be put through a range of motion that has already been performed, particularly looking for hyperextension compared with the opposite side **(Fig. 6-17)**. When putting the knee through a range of motion with the patient supine and 90 degrees of flexion of both hips and knees, the physician can appreciate any posterior sag of the tibia that may be

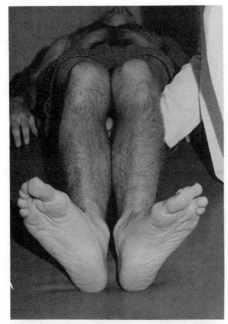

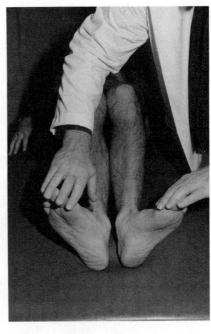

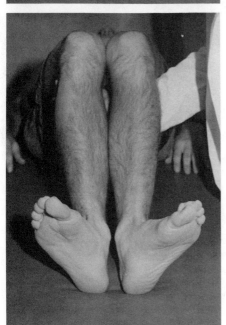

Figure 6-23.
A, This demonstrates assessment of external rotation of the tibia using the medial border of the foot, actively performed by the patient. If abnormal on one side, posterolateral instability is possible. B, This is the same phenomenon performed passively by the examiner. C, This is the same testing done at 90 degrees of knee flexion, which is more in keeping with both a posterolateral and posterior cruciate deficiency if positive.

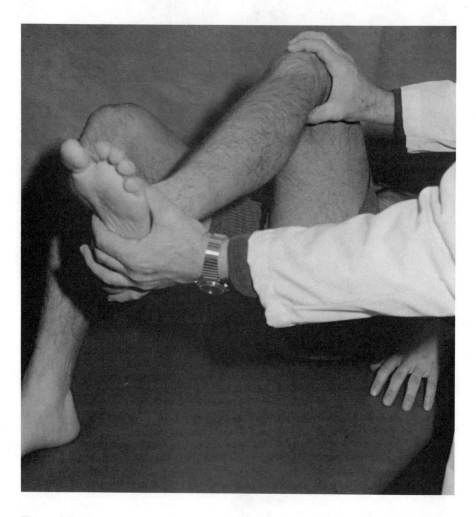

Figure 6-24.
Reverse pivot shifting is performed by bringing the knee from a flexed position with a valgus axial load and the tibia externally rotated. As the knee approaches approximately 40 degrees of extension, a pivoting phenomena brings the tibia to the neutral position.

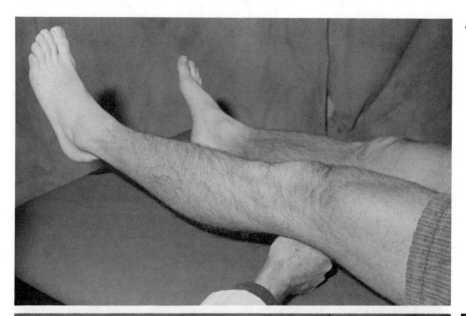

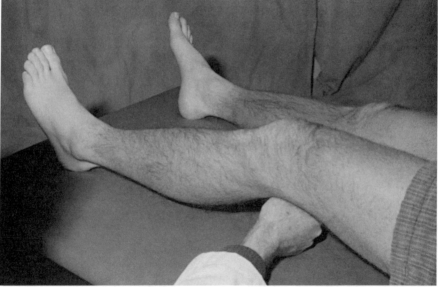

Figure 6-25.
A, Dynamic anterior cruciate testing is helpful in the acute stage. This demonstrates active extension of the knee with the examiner's fist placed under the popliteal fossa. B, As the patient brings the knee actively down to the tabletop and relaxes, the examiner should look for posterior subluxation of the tibia, indicating a reverse Lachman maneuver.

Stability (Laxity) Assessment   197

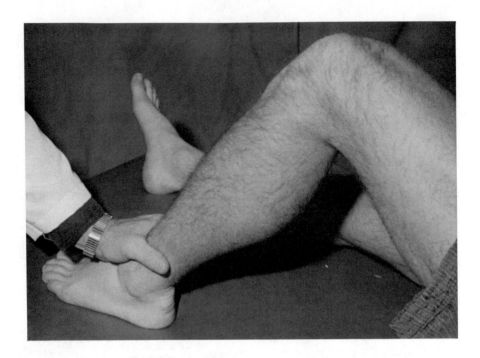

Figure 6-26.
Quadriceps active or dynamic resistance testing for the posterior cruciate is performed with the knee flexed at 90 degrees and the patient pushing distally on the examining table while the examiner offers resistance. In this position with a posterior cruciate deficiency, the tibial plateau is pulled forward by the contraction of the quadriceps.

present (Fig. 6-27). This may be augmented by pushing posteriorly on the proximal tibia with careful comparison with the opposite side.

In the fully extended position, various methods can be applied to assess valgus and varus instability, which can be determined by grasping or buttressing the lateral aspect of the knee with one hand and grasping the heel and ankle with the opposite hand and applying a valgus (Fig. 6-2, B) or varus (Fig. 6-18, A) stress. It can also be performed by putting the foot in the armpit and palpating the joint lines on each side while applying a valgus and varus stress. Another method that might be useful in the patient who is in pain is to rest the thigh on the table and drop the part distal to the knee over the edge of the table when applying valgus and varus

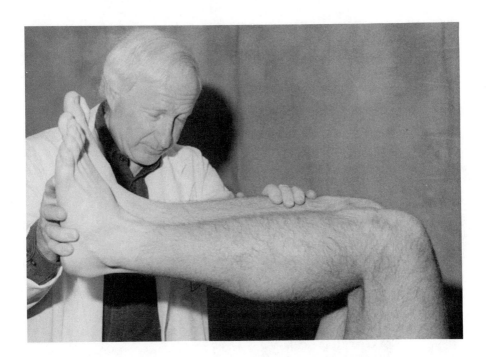

Figure 6-27.
This is the position to demonstrate a posterior sag, where the knees are flexed up to 90 degrees and compared. Slight posterior pressure can elicit any sag that might be present.

stresses **(Fig. 6-2, A).** Subtleties abound and each examiner has a preference as to the best method of eliciting the maximum laxity that may be present. The knee is again tested at approximately 30 degrees of flexion with both valgus and varus instability. The examiner can sit on the edge of the examining table and, laying the involved extremity across his lap to achieve relaxation, apply a varus stress to document varus laxity **(Fig. 6-18, B).** Similarly, a Lachman maneuver or an anterior drawer at 20 to 30 degrees of flexion is performed to assess anterior cruciate deficiency **(Fig. 6-19).** This can be difficult to perform, particularly in patients with large extremities, yet is the most reliable test for an acute anterior cruciate ligament disruption. Not only is the excursion or translation considered with Lachman testing, but also the end point as to whether soft or firm. A firm end point with a click in an acute knee injury almost precludes the diagnosis of an acute anterior cruciate ligament disruption. In patients with large legs, placing the examiner's knee under the distal thigh, putting the knee in slight flexion for relaxation purposes, and then performing a Lachman maneuver can be performed without having to grasp both distal thigh and proximal tibia with the examiner's hands, described as the Hawkins maneuver **(Fig. 6-28)**.

At 90 degrees of flexion with the examiner sitting on the patient's foot, anterior and posterior drawer testing can be performed in the neutral position **(Fig. 6-5)**. Anterior drawering is also performed with the lower extremity externally and internally rotated, not maximally, but just short of full rotation. Similarly, with the hips flexed 90 degrees and the knee flexed 90 degrees,

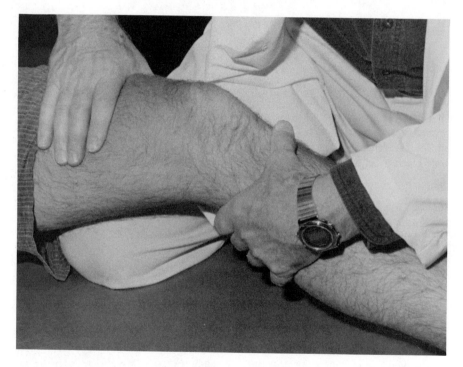

Figure 6-28.
In the acute setting, particularly in a large patient, a positive Lachman test, if present, is sometimes difficult to elicit. Placing the examiner's knee under the patient's thigh at about 30 degrees of flexion relaxes the patient's hamstrings, enabling the examiner to pull the tibia forward, eliciting a Lachman sign if it is present. This test is particularly helpful in the acute situation.

the physician can visually observe a posterior sag, and with posterior drawering this can be augmented if present (**Fig. 6-27**). If an element of varus instability and posterior drawering is present, examining for posterolateral instability may be prudent at this point. Sliding the thumbs from the femur to the tibial plateau in the 90 degree flexed position should feel the thumb abut against the tibial plateau. The absence of this feeling is the thumb sign, suggestive of posterior cruciate insufficiency (**Fig. 6-29**).

The patient can then be assessed for anterior cruciate deficiency with the various pivot shift maneuvers. The MacIntosh maneuver applies a valgus stress axial load with the foot usually in neutral rotation, progressing from full extension into the flexed position (**Fig. 6-20**). The hypothenar eminence of the examiner's

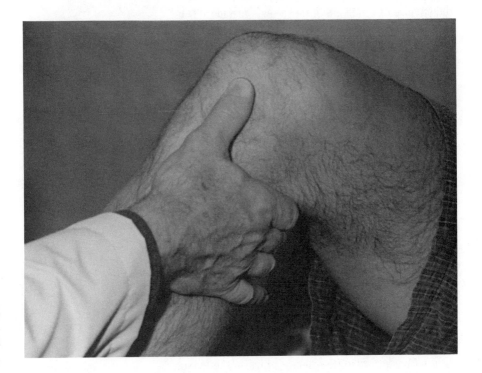

Figure 6-29.
When the thumb is brought down from the femoral condyles to the tibial plateau in the presence of a posterior cruciate tear with a posterior sag, the thumb does not abut the tibial plateau but slides by. This is known as the thumb sign.

hand is placed over the fibular head to apply this valgus loading. An appreciation of reduction is the classical pivot shift. The Losee maneuver is a subluxation occurrence from flexion into extension, elicited with similar valgus and axial loading with the tibia in various degrees of rotation (Fig. 6-21). During these two tests, the examiner should ask if the patient appreciates this as part of the symptom complex. A positive answer strongly suggests anterior cruciate ligament (ACL) deficiency as at least part of the patient's problem.

The flexion/rotation drawer testing consists of a reverse Lachman test as the first component, followed by valgus and axial loading for the pivoting phenomenon (Fig. 6-22). Other forms of pivoting are then applied, such as the jerk test described by Hughston. These tests and their various modifications allow the physician to appreciate any pivoting, either of a subluxation or a reduction pattern. Some of these tests are more reliable in acute injuries, others more helpful in chronic injuries. Some are more effective in the presence of pain. Understanding how to perform different methods of pivoting help elicit the diagnosis of ACL deficiency.

Posterolateral Instability

Hughston has described two tests for posterolateral instability and subsequent modifications have evolved. His first test consists of lifting the big toe and noting any excessive recurvatum in the posterolateral aspect of the knee as the tibia drops off. This test has not proven as helpful as assessment of excessive external rotation of the tibial tubercle manifest by distal tibial rotation at 30, 60, and 90 degrees of flexion (Fig. 6-23, A, B, C). This can be measured supine or prone, and is usually documented with the medial border of the foot, but care must be taken to consider spurious ankle rotation. The test can be performed either actively by the patient or passively by the examiner. If a posterior drawer occurs at 90 degrees of flexion, the tibia can be noted to rotate externally farther than the opposite normal side with a drop off posteriorly of the tibia relative to the femur. Part of this symptom complex is the associated reverse pivot shift. This shifting occurs when taking the knee from flexion to extension, commencing at 90 degrees of flexion and applying a valgus and axial load with the distal tibia externally rotated **(Fig. 6-24)**. The reverse pivot has the tibia come from a displaced posterolateral position to neutral and can easily be mistaken for a pivot shift. In fact, it can be found in an ACL-deficient knee so that both a reverse and a true pivot may be present. Some recent investigators believe that a previously described Grade I pivot shift in some physiologically lax knees represents a reverse pivot phenomenon. With posterolateral instability, a mild grade of varus instability at 30 degrees of flexion almost always exists.

Dynamic Instability Assessment

Dynamic testing for ligamentous instability is frequently helpful. Dynamic ACL deficiency can be demonstrated by placing a fist under the patient's knee on the examining table, and asking the patient to extend the extremity and then slowly lower it onto the tabletop **(Fig. 6-25, A, B)**. Often as the heel strikes the tabletop and the patient relaxes the quadriceps, the tibia appears to posteriorly sublux, which in actual fact is moving from its anteriorly subluxed position to neutral. This represents a reverse Lachman maneuver. Similarly, the quadriceps resistance test for posterior cruciate ligament deficiency is performed with the knee flexed at 90 degrees, the foot laying flat on the tabletop, and with the patient pushing the ankle forward against resistance from the examiner **(Fig. 6-26)**. In the posterior cruciate ligament deficient knee, this quadriceps contraction pulls the tibia forward from a posteriorly displaced position.

Patellofemoral Instability

Forgetting to examine the patellofemoral joint when examining the knee is common. When examining the patellofemoral joint, the physician may combine various specialized testing with instability assessment. Laxity assessment of the patella consists of translating it laterally and medially and assessing its excursion **(Fig. 6-30)**. The patella can be divided into quadrants and an estimate of which quadrant passes the apex of the opposing femoral condyle. For example, if the physician applies a lateral stress and the patella is felt to go over the apex of the lateral femoral condyle, it

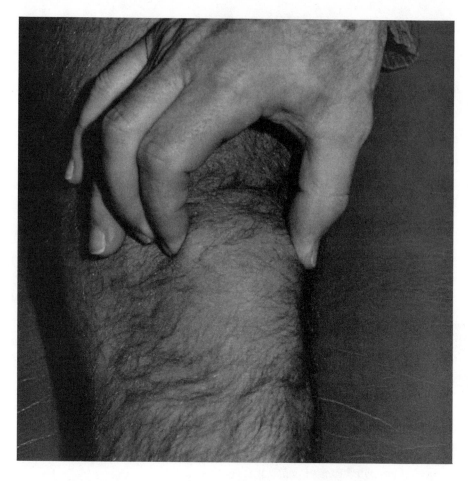

Figure 6-30.
Laxity assessment of the patella consists of translating it laterally and medially and assessing its excursion relative to the opposing femoral condyle.

would go at least into the third quadrant (from 50% to 75%). The examiner also looks for an apprehension sign suggestive of patellar instability by stressing the patella laterally in both neutral and 30 degrees of flexion **(Fig. 6-7)**.

During examination of the patella with stressing, the physician should note any pain, reproduction of symptomatology, and feeling of crepitus. To augment this crepitus, the examiner can apply direct pressure over the patella, forcing it against the femoral condyle. This Osmond-Clarke test often reproduces pain, frequently with an appreciation of crepitus. This test has modifications, such as pushing the patella distally into the groove, noting any crepitus and pain, and then asking

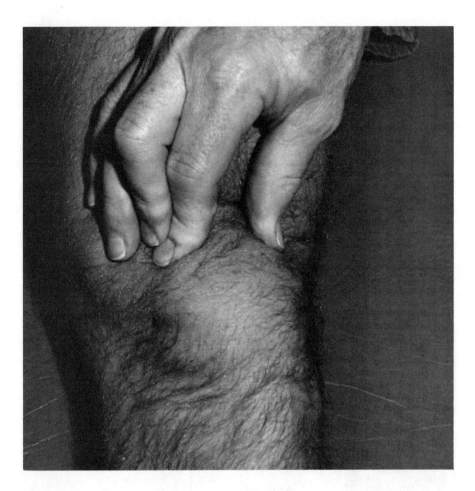

Figure 6-31.

A modification of the Osmond-Clarke test consists of pushing the patella distally into the groove in the extended position and, asking the patient to contract the quadriceps, noting any reproduction of crepitus and pain.

the patient to contract his quadriceps while the examiner loads the patella distally to see if this increases pain or causes any of his symptoms **(Fig. 6-31)**. This grinding test also has various modifications. Crepitus is perhaps more efficiently felt in the sitting position as the patient actively extends the knee from the flexed position with the examiner holding his palm over the patella **(Fig. 4-65)**. These are not aspects of instability of the patella, but obviously important components to assessment of the patella and are described here for completeness.

In the sitting and supine positions the examiner must note the height of the patella and compare it to the opposite side, which is particularly important in the postoperative painful knee when the patella sometimes is pulled inferiorly from infrapatellar contracture. Tenderness over the patellar tendon suggests patellar tendinitis or jumper's knee **(Fig. 6-32)**.

In the patient who has anterior knee pain, patellar tracking should be observed as the patient flexes and extends. In the sitting position, movement in the patellar groove can be assessed. For example, a J-sign,

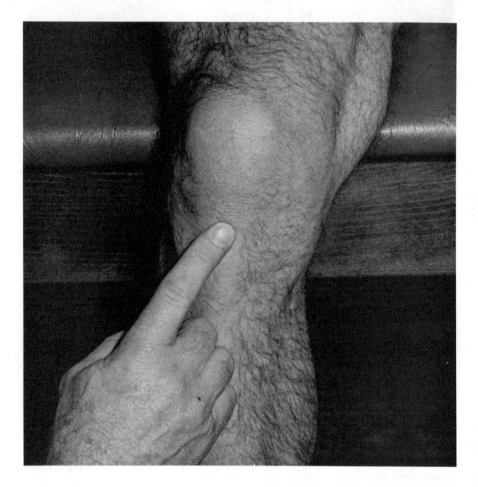

Figure 6-32.
Assessing the patellofemoral complex and the patellar tendon in the sitting position is important. Noting the height of the patella relative to the opposite side and eliciting any areas of tenderness, suggestive of patellar tendinitis, are also important.

where the patella jumps laterally as the knee is extended, may be present, which suggests maltracking.

The Q-angle, which is normally 7 to 10 degrees, can usually best be assessed standing, but it can also be documented sitting or supine.

Ankle Instability

Assessment of ankle instability consists predominantly of two maneuvers. The first is a lateral tilt or inversion stress; the second is an anterior drawer stress **(Fig. 6-33)**. In the acute setting, feeling lateral ligamentous instability when stressing with an inversion stress is nearly impossible because of pain and

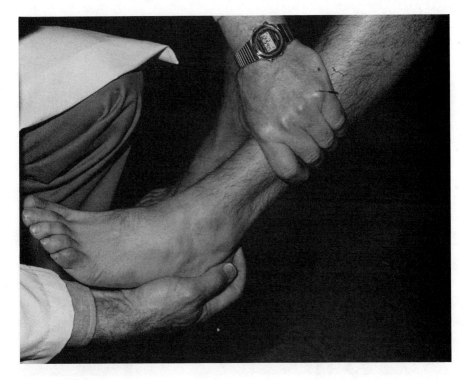

Figure 6-33.
An anterior drawer test can be performed to assess ligamentous instability by positioning the ankle at approximately 20 degrees of flexion, holding the tibia back with one hand, and pulling forward on the ankle mortise with the opposite hand. Excess excursion, which is often associated with a clunk, may suggest instability.

swelling. In the chronic setting, lateral instability can sometimes be appreciated. With the ankle flexed approximately 20 degrees, sometimes an anterior drawer can be elicited by feeling the talus move forward in the ankle mortise. The anterior drawer sign may be associated with a palpable or audible clunk as the talus moves forward. Both tests are probably best performed in the sitting position with the ankle free to be more easily manipulated.

Elbow Instability

Varus and valgus instability of the elbow is difficult to appreciate. It can be rather subtle and requires practice and experience on the part of the examiner. Valgus

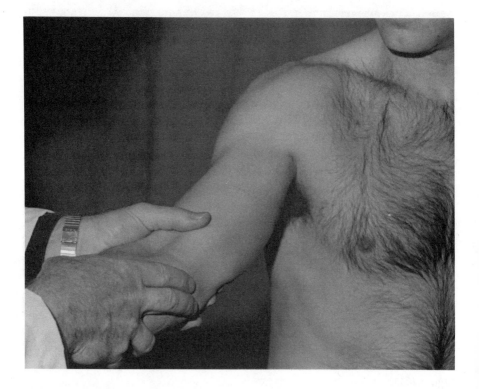

Figure 6-34.
Valgus instability of the elbow is determined by placing the index and long finger over the medial joint line and applying a valgus stress at approximately 15 to 20 degrees of elbow flexion. This must be compared with the opposite side and can be a difficult determination.

and varus stresses should be applied at both 0 and approximately 30 degrees of flexion, while controlling rotation (Fig. 6-34). In an acute elbow injury, this assessment is doubly difficult. Valgus overload, particularly in an athlete who throws, can lead to instability and should be carefully documented in such individuals. Unfortunately, its subtleness can often confuse the inexperienced examiner.

Thumb Metacarpophalangeal Instability

The gamekeeper's thumb or disruption of the ulnar collateral ligament of the thumb can be documented on physical examination (Fig. 6-3). If acute due to pain and swelling, the diagnosis can be difficult; if chronic, it is easier. A radial deviation of the distal segment is determined by an angular stress applied in both neutral and at 30 degrees of flexion, noting increase in angulation compared to the opposite side. If the injury is acute, 30 degrees of angulation greater than the normal side indicates complete disruption of the ulnar collateral ligament; 15 to 30 degrees, a partial disruption; and less than 15 degrees, a questionable diagnosis of ligamentous involvement. The physician should examine at not only 30 degrees of flexion, but also at 0 degrees in that instability at both angles may suggest involvement of the volar plate. As with knee instability, a soft rather than firm end point is an important finding.

Hip Instability

Assessment of instability of the hip is generally not applied to patients who have hip pain and osteoarthritis unless following arthroplasty. Following reduction of a dislocated hip in an adult or when examining a newborn, certain instability tests should be performed. Following reduction of a dislocated hip in the operating room, the examiner should flex, internally rotate, and apply a posterior stress to see if the hip easily redislocates again, suggestive of a posterior rim fracture allowing this instability. In the newborn, documentation of hip instability should be part of every examination.

Ortolani's sign consists of reduction of a dislocated hip when the hip is abducted (Fig. 6-35). Barlow's modification of Ortolani's sign consists of abduction and adduction of the hip, using the thumb and fingers

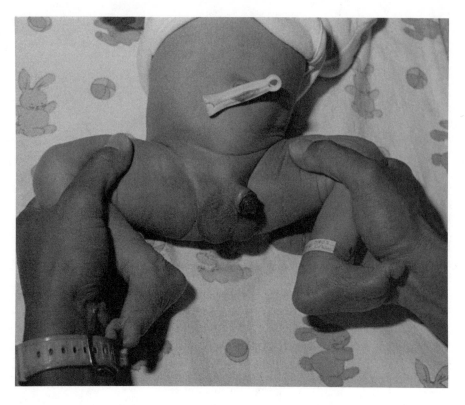

Figure 6-35.
Ortolani's sign consists of abducting a newborn's hip and feeling a clunk, representing a reduction from a dislocated position.

attempting to lever the femoral head out of and into the socket **(Fig. 6-36)**. Similarly, in the flexed and internally rotated position, a telescoping stress may result in a feeling of the femoral head riding over the rim of the acetabulum with a pushing maneuver and reducing with a pulling maneuver.

Summary

These represent some of the instability patterns seen in various joints of the body, in both the acute and chronic setting. In order to appreciate these instability patterns, particularly in the presence of pain, the physician must help the patient relax. Assessing joint instability is easier and more reliable with a totally relaxed, anesthetized patient. In certain circumstances, the anesthesiologist might be reminded to provide muscle relaxation when examining for instability. In the awake patient, if the physician does not convince the patient to relax his hamstrings, anterior

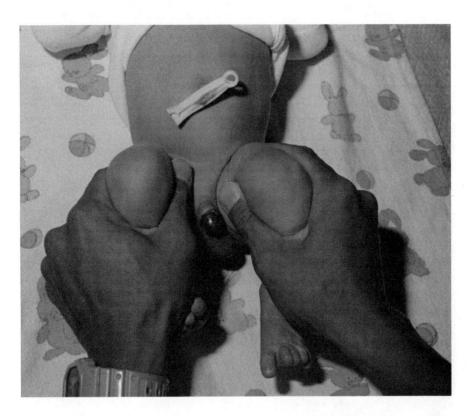

Figure 6-36.
Barlow's modification of Ortolani's sign represents a levering attempt to sublux the head into or out of the socket.

drawering or translation at 90 degrees of flexion of the tibia on the femur may never be appreciated **(Fig. 6-5)**. Postoperatively, signs of prosthetic looseness following total hip and total knee replacements suggest instability, not so much of the joint but of the prosthetic components. This relates to clunking and abnormal sensations felt by the patient upon certain stress testing and range of motion.

In the acute setting, a patient can present with an obvious locked dislocation. This commonly occurs, for example, in a patient who has been exposed to trauma, resulting in an anterior dislocation of the shoulder. Such a patient presents with the arm cradled across the abdomen supported with the opposite extremity, obviously in great pain and refusing any movement **(Fig. 6-37)**. A patient who has a dislocated hip may present with the knee flexed, shortened, and internally rotated **(Fig. 6-38)**. A patient may present following a direct blow to the tip of the shoulder with a prominent outer

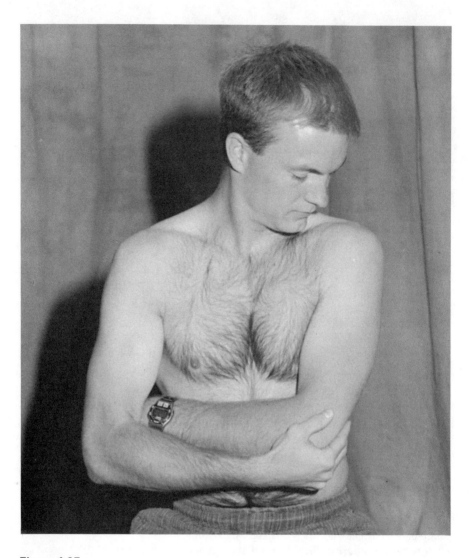

Figure 6-37.
This patient presents with an obvious locked dislocation,
which is common in those exposed to trauma.

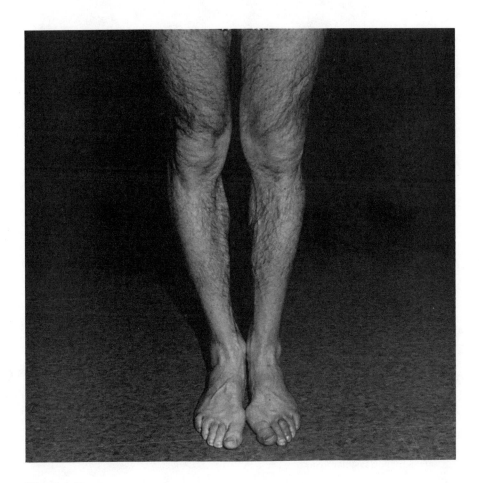

Figure 6-38.
A patient with a dislocated hip presents with the involved extremity shortened and internally rotated, lying across the opposite extremity.

clavicle, an acromioclavicular dislocation (**Fig. 6-39**). These acute presentations documented on physical examination present differently than the patterns previously described for various instability patterns. They nevertheless warrant discussion in appreciation of joint instability.

Documentation of Instability

Documentation of ligamentous instability in various joints of the body has already been discussed. Angular stresses can be documented in angulation or in millimeters of opening affecting the joint (**Fig. 6-2, B**).

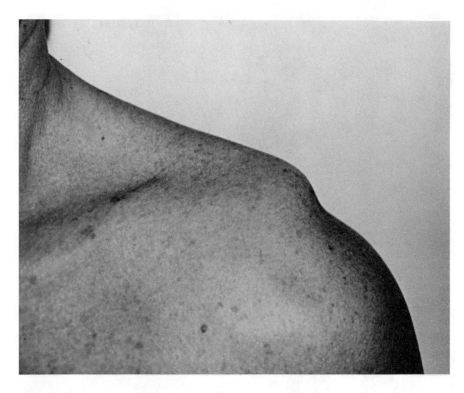

Figure 6-39.
Patients may present following a direct blow to the tip of the shoulder with a prominent outer clavicle, suggestive of a complete acromioclavicular dislocation.

Translation similarly can be documented in terms of millimeters of displacement compared to the opposite side. The examiner must keep in mind that these assessments need be compared and objectively classified relative to the opposite extremity if it is normal. If the opposite extremity is not normal, then the examiner needs to estimate relative to what would be normal for that situation, considering factors such as age and sex. Apprehension cannot be objectively graded but can be subjectively graded in terms of its degree such as mild, moderate, or severe (**Fig. 6-8, A, B, C**).

Chapter

7 Special Tests

A separate section of the examination should be reserved for special tests. At this part of the examination, looking back and ensuring that all appropriate tests as they relate to specific parts have been performed is vital. Throughout the examination, perhaps the physician has performed some of these tests but forgotten others. For example, an impingement sign possibly would have been elicited when the examiner performed range of motion of the shoulder (**Figs. 7-1, 7-2**). In a patient who has a painful arc, the examiner would have performed that test when the shoulder was abducted (**Fig. 7-3**). If these tests have not been performed, the examiner can perform them now. If physicians do not have a section for special tests, having completed the examination, they may well forget to do tests such as McMurray's test in the knee (**Fig. 7-4**), which is indicative of meniscal pathology, or a Trendelenburg's test of the hip (**Fig. 7-5**), which is suggestive of hip pathology. Looking at each area and analyzing some of these special tests is, therefore, prudent.

Text continued on p. 220.

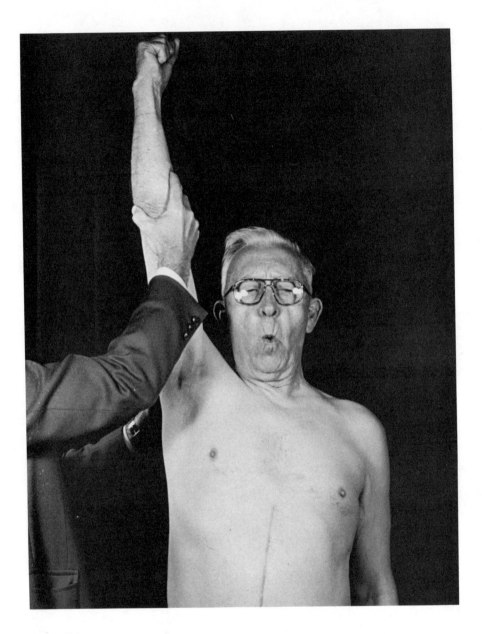

Figure 7-1.
This demonstrates the impingement sign, which elicits pain
by forcibly jamming the tuberosity of a forward flexed arm
against the anterior acromion.

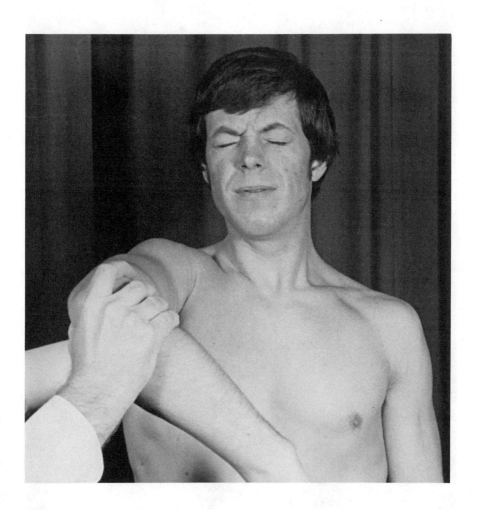

Figure 7-2.
This demonstrates an impingement sign by forcibly internally
rotating the 90 degree elevated and forward flexed arm.

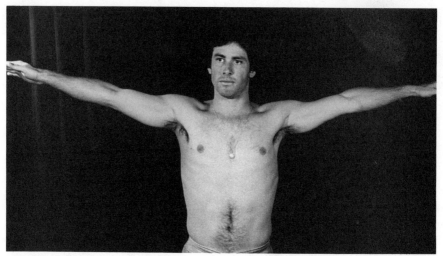

Figure 7-3.
In a patient with a painful arc, the patient abducts the shoulder, which may be painful and is often augmented with resistance. This is another impingement sign.

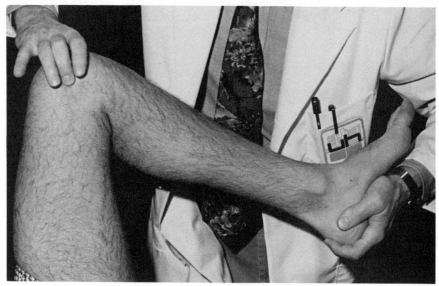

Figure 7-4.
One special test to assess a meniscus tear in the knee is McMurray's test. It consists of rotating the flexed knee between 90 degrees and full flexion, eliciting a clunk from the appropriate medial or lateral compartment.

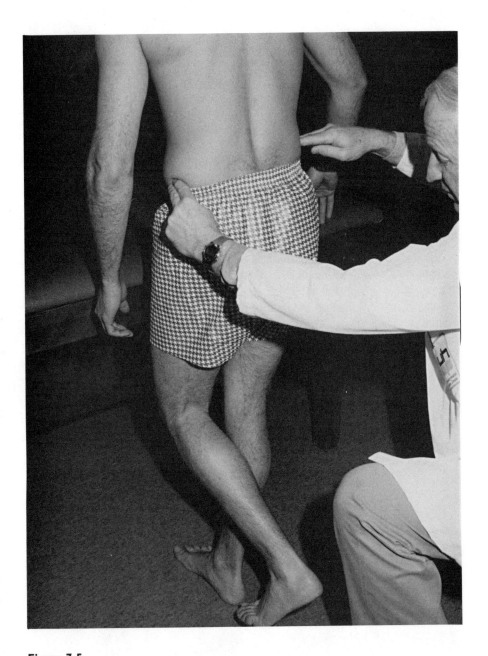

Figure 7-5.
In the chapter on Special Tests, Trendelenburg's test of the hip suggestive of gluteus maximus weakness and hip disease may not have been performed. A positive Trendelenburg sign demonstrated here shows the left hip dropping when it is unweighted.

Cervical Spine

Special tests to consider in the cervical spine consist of compression **(Fig. 7-6, A)** and distraction testing **(Fig. 7-6, B)**, Spurling's test **(Fig. 7-6, C)**, and testing for Lhermitte's sign. Frequently, patients who have pain emanating from the cervical spine with or without root involvement may find relief with distraction of the head in the slightly flexed position **(Fig. 7-6, B)**. Standing from behind, the examiner can cup the patient's head at the angles of the jaw, gently lifting upward, thereby decompressing the posterior facet joints and opening the foramina to relieve pain from cervical spine and root pathology. Similarly, in the slightly extended position, the examiner can percuss the top of the head to increase the neck pain, sometimes with pain radiating into a root distribution. This represents positive compression testing. Spurling's test consists of axially loading the laterally flexed and rotated cervical spine, causing pain. This is a nonspecific test, suggestive of some pathology in the neck. Lhermitte's sign is a rather dramatic Tinel sign produced by direct percussion over an area of compression of the cervical spine posteriorly, causing an electric shock–like sensation to radiate into the legs and arms.

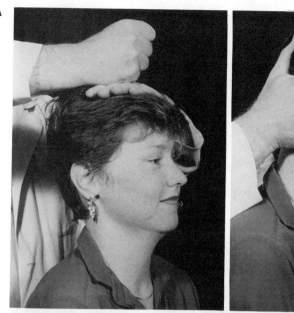
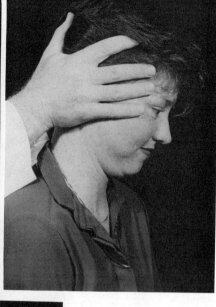
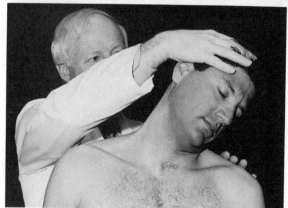

Figure 7-6.

A, Compression testing of the cervical spine, eliciting pain in the cervical spine or radiating down the extremities, is demonstrated. It is suggestive of cervical disk disease and/or root involvement, the latter particularly so with radiation. B, Distraction testing relieves pain in the cervical spine and/or radiating pain into the extremities and is suggestive of degenerative cervical disk disease perhaps with root involvement. C, This demonstrates Spurling's test, which produces neck pain when the neck is laterally flexed, rotated, and compressed.

Shoulder

Special tests relating to the shoulder that may or may not have been performed consist of the various impingement signs **(Figs. 7-1, 7-2)**, painful arc **(Fig. 7-3)**, Speed's test **(Fig. 7-7)**, and Yergason's test **(Fig. 7-8)**, indicative of bicipital pathology, and perhaps some of the instability maneuvers that should have already been assessed.

Three described methods of assessing impingement in the shoulder exist. The first consists of forcibly elevating the arm against the anterior acromion in the fully elevated position reproducing pain, suggesting subacromial impingement **(Fig. 7-1)**. The second test consists of forcibly internally rotating the 90-degree

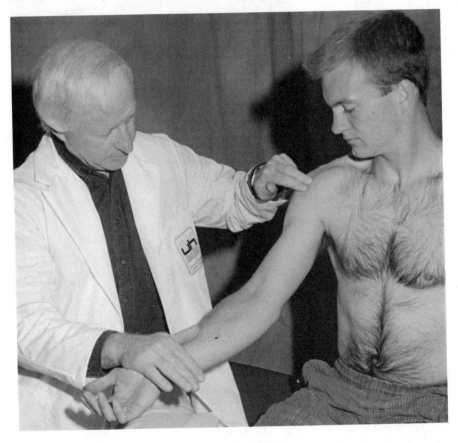

Figure 7-7.
Speed's test reproduces pain in the area of the bicipital groove, produced with resisted elevation of the slightly flexed arm.

forward flexed arm in neutral rotation, again reproducing pain by jamming the greater tuberosity against the leading edge of the coracoacromial ligament (**Fig. 7-2**). A painful arc in the coronal plane maximum at 90 degrees of active elevation is also suggestive of impingement (**Fig. 7-3**). This may be augmented with resistance at this 90 degree abducted position (**Fig. 7-9**). Speed's test consists of a positive reproduction of pain in the area of the bicipital tendon with resisted elevation of the arm at about 30 degrees of elbow flexion (**Fig. 7-7**). A positive Yergason's test consists of this same pain in the area of the bicipital groove, produced with resisted supination, the arm at the side and the elbow flexed 90 degrees (**Fig. 7-8**). Forced

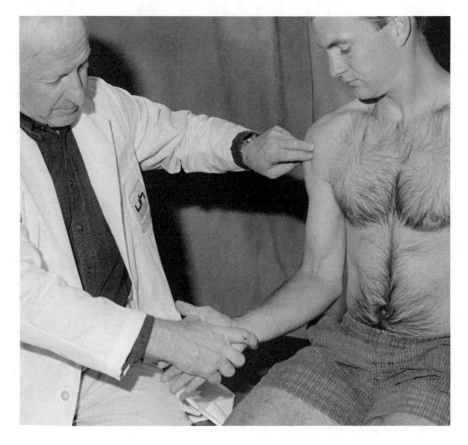

Figure 7-8.
Yergason's test reproduces pain in the area of the bicipital groove with resisted supination of the forearm with the arm at the side.

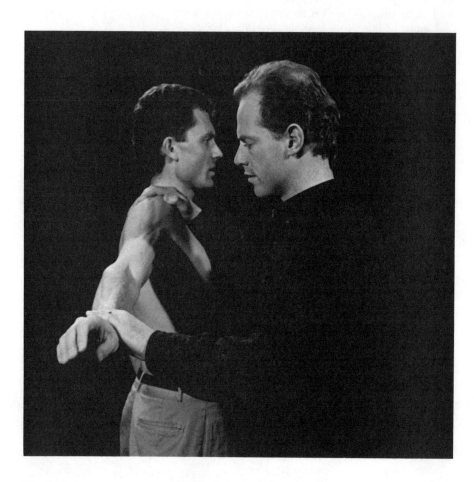

Figure 7-9.
Resisted abduction in the coronal plane often augments the
presence of an impingement sign or the painful arc.

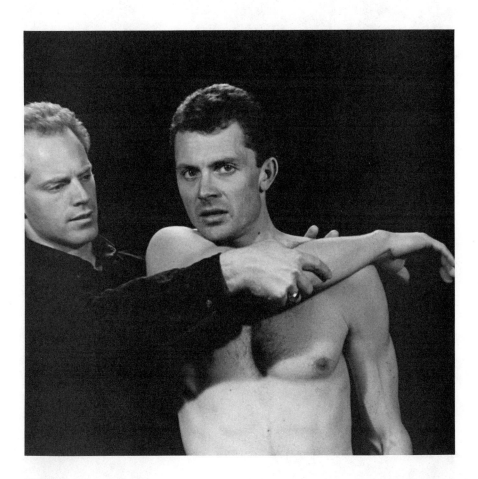

Figure 7-10.
Another special test in the shoulder forces crossed arm abduction producing pain, suggestive of acromioclavicular pathology.

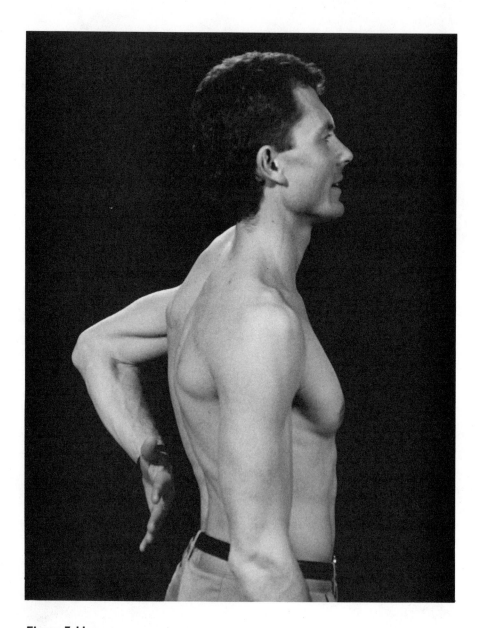

Figure 7-11.
The lift-off test is performed by asking the patient to lift the
hand away from the small of the back. Inability to do this may
suggest a subscapularis rupture.

crossed arm adduction producing pain is suggestive of acromioclavicular pathology **(Fig. 7-10)**.

Christian Gerber has described a test that suggests a complete disruption of the subscapularis tendon, known as the lift-off test **(Fig. 7-11)**. This is performed by asking the patient to place his hand behind his back and lift it away from the back. An ability to perform the lift-off test indicates an intact subscapularis, while an inability to perform the lift-off test may suggest a subscapularis disruption. Unfortunately, however, this might be positive in a very painful shoulder and in a shoulder with adhesive capsulitis.

Patients with a snapping scapula demonstrate palpable or audible crepitus with movement of the scapula on the chest wall. This can be magnified by auscultation using a stethoscope or placing a microphone over the area. Scapular winging can be elicited by having the patient push against a wall **(Fig. 7-12)**.

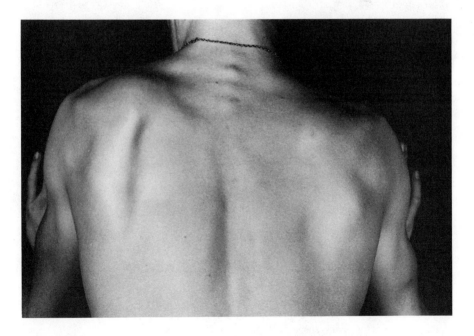

Figure 7-12.
Scapular winging can be elicited by having the patient push against a wall.

Elbow

Pain with resisted dorsiflexion of the wrist referred to the lateral aspect of the elbow may suggest a diagnosis of tennis elbow **(Fig. 7-13)**. Similarly, pain with resisted palmar flexion of the wrist referred to the medial aspect of the elbow may suggest medial epicondylitis or flexor tendinosis. Testing is also done for posterolateral instability of the elbow by a maneuver described as a pivot shift test of the elbow.

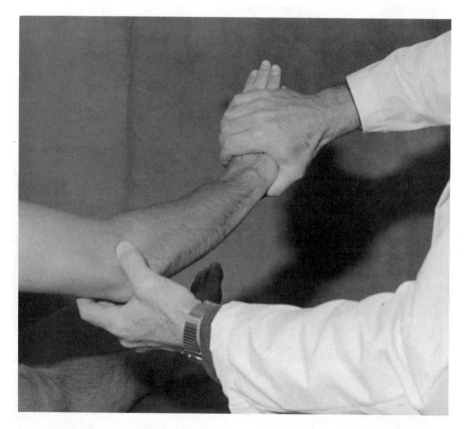

Figure 7-13.
Pain with resisted dorsiflexion of the wrist referred to the lateral aspect of the elbow, suggests tennis elbow. Similarly, patients with lateral epicondylitis have marked tenderness over the lateral epicondyle at the insertion of the extensor tendons.

Hand and Wrist

Finkelstein's test, suggestive of tendinitis of the thumb abductors, consists of forcing the flexed and adducted thumb across the palm, stretching the tendons and causing pain (**Fig. 7-14**). Phalen's test consists of forcibly flexing the wrist, reproducing pain and paresthesias in the distribution of the median nerve, suggestive of a carpal tunnel syndrome (**Fig. 7-15**). Similarly, Tinel's test should be performed at the wrist (**Fig. 7-16**) and elbow (**Fig. 7-17**), looking for median or ulnar entrapment. Tinel's test consists of percussion over the nerve reproducing pain and dysesthesia in the distribution of the nerve, indicative of entrapment or neuropathy. The reader should refer to specialized texts for tests related to hand pathology.

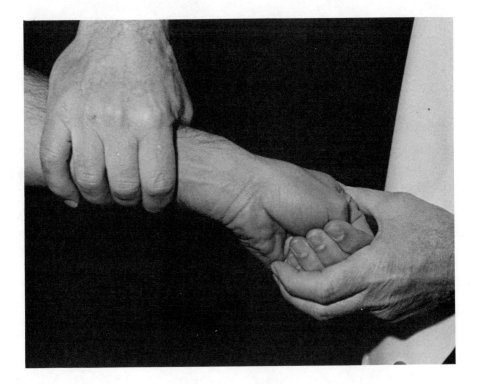

Figure 7-14.
Finkelstein's test suggests tendinitis of the thumb abductors and is performed by forcing the flexed and adducted thumb across the palm, stretching the tendons and causing pain.

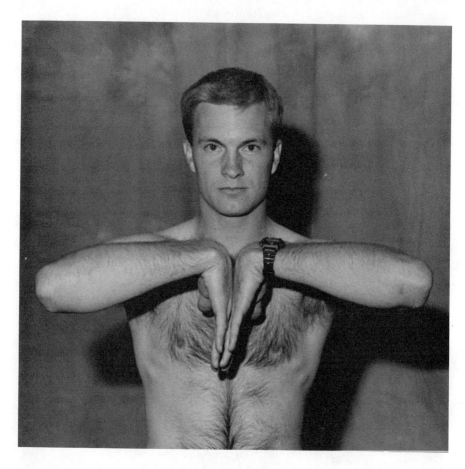

Figure 7-15.
Phalen's test has the patient forcibly flexing the wrists together, reproducing pain and paresthesias in the distribution of the median nerve, suggestive of a carpal tunnel syndrome.

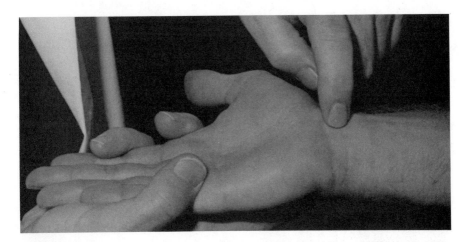

Figure 7-16.
Tinel's test, performed at the wrist, may produce paresthesias and pain in the distribution of the median nerve.

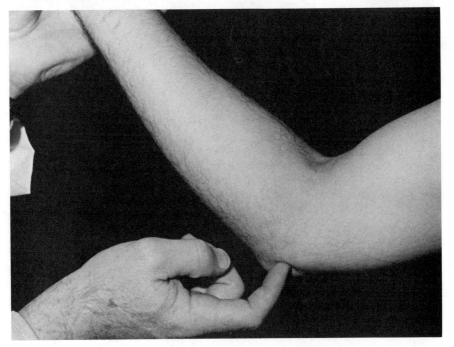

Figure 7-17.
Tinel's sign suggests nerve irritation. The presence of Tinel's sign at the elbow—the test is performed by gently tapping on the nerve—causes radiating pain into the distribution of that nerve and is suggestive of some form of neuropathy.

Thoracic Outlet Tests

Thoracic outlet tests are discussed in the chapter on Vascularity, but they consist of specialized testing to document a thoracic outlet. These consist of Adson's test **(Fig. 7-18)**, the attention position, and the hyperabduction maneuver. In all of these tests, a diminished pulse is considered positive. Perhaps the best maneuver for thoracic outlet is a provocative test, which consists of having the patient elevate the arms above the horizontal position and repetitively open and close the hands, thereby reproducing symptoms in the distal extremities **(Fig. 7-19)**.

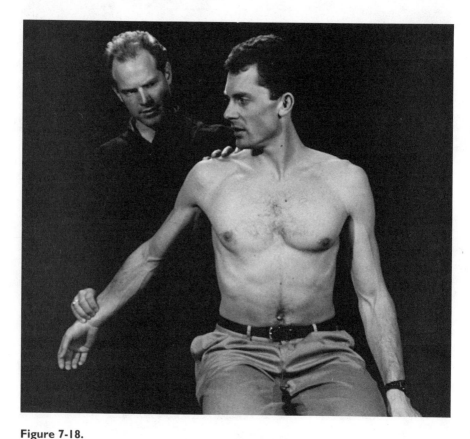

Figure 7-18.
Adson's test is demonstrated, eliciting a diminished pulse, with the arm extended and the head turned toward the same side. Sides are compared and are more meaningful if different.

Special Neurological Tests

In the chapter on Neurological Examination, tests that relate to the neurological system would have been performed. Tests such as Tinel's test, Lhermitte's sign, and Phalen's test have already been described.

Hip

With regard to newborns, specialized tests consisting of Ortolani's sign and Barlow's modification of Ortolani's sign to assess stability have already been de-

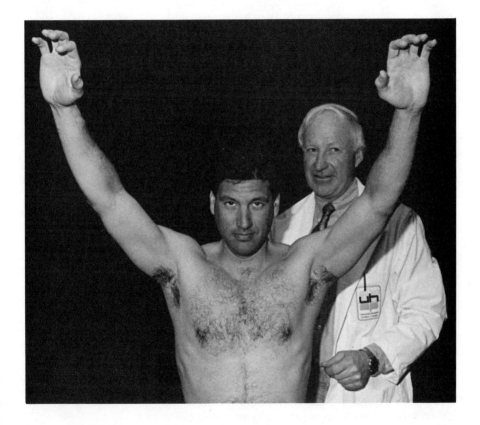

Figure 7-19.
Perhaps the best maneuver for thoracic outlet is a provocative test, which consists of having the patient elevate the arms above the horizontal position and repetitively open and close the hands. Reproducing symptoms in the distal extremities suggests thoracic outlet syndrome.

scribed (see Figs. 6-35, 6-36). The Thomas test is described under range of motion and is particularly important in the adult with osteoarthritis (see Fig. 4-54). Often, the physician may have forgotten to do a Trendelenburg test (Fig. 7-5); however, it may be performed at this time in this section of special testing. The Trendelenburg test is performed with the examiner behind the patient, observing any dropping off of the iliac crest on the normal side as the patient stands on the affected extremity. Ely's test consists of observing elevation of the buttock in a prone patient when the knee is flexed. In a child with cerebral palsy this suggests rectus femoris rather than psoas contracture causing the hip flexion deformity. Ober's test assesses an abduction contracture common in the past when polio was prevalent. With the hip extended and the knee flexed, contracture of the band would make bringing the hip into the adducted position impossible.

Knee

Special tests of the knee consist of maneuvers such as McMurray's test (Fig. 7-4), Apley's distraction and compression test (Fig. 7-20), Wilson's test, and the Osmond-Clarke test. Some of these have already been described. Again, performing McMurray's test in the knee might easily have been forgotten unless it was done during the range of motion testing. McMurray's test suggests a piece of meniscus lodging or becoming freed between the femoral and tibial condyles with various rotational maneuvers with the knee flexed and extended between 90 and 140 degrees (Fig. 7-4). It reproduces an audible or palpable clunk emanating from the appropriate compartment. Apley's testing distinguishes osteoarthritic from ligamentous pathology causing knee pain. In the prone position with the knee flexed 90 degrees, pain with rotational movements and compression suggests osteoarthritis; with distraction, ligamentous pain. A positive result in Wilson's test causes pain resulting from forcibly externally rotating the flexed knee, driving the anterior cruciate against an osteochondritis dissecans lesion on the medial aspect of the lateral femoral condyle. The Osmond-Clarke test has already been described (Fig. 7-21). For a posterior cruciate tear and a posterior

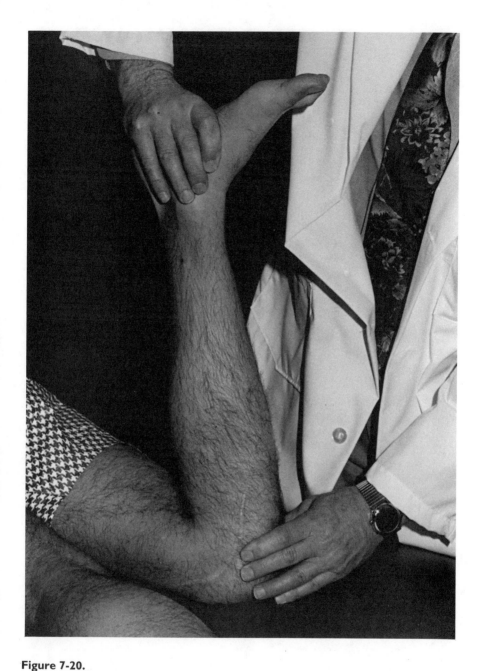

Figure 7-20.
Apley's distraction and compression test distinguishes between pain produced from meniscus and ligamentous pathology. Compressing the flexed knee with the patient in the prone
position eliciting pain suggests meniscal pathology.

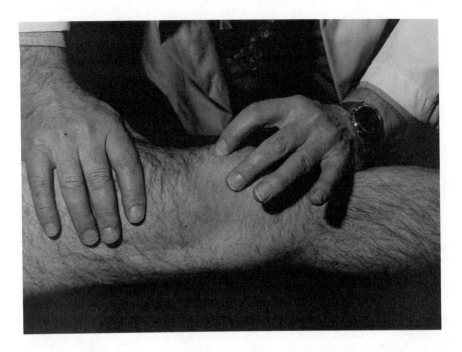

Figure 7-21.
This maneuver demonstrates compression of the patella against the underlying femoral condyles and groove, producing pain suggestive of patellofemoral pathology. Various modifications of this Osmond-Clarke test exist.

sag, the thumb sign has been described and consists of pulling the thumb down from the patella to the tibial plateau. Normally, the thumb abuts the tibial plateau. If the tibia is posteriorly displaced, the thumb does not abut the plateau (see Fig. 6-29).

Chapter

8   Measurements

Throughout this discussion, objective documentation has been stressed. Measurements provide that objective documentation, and a separate chapter here precludes omitting this important segment of the physical examination. Measurements accurately document what may be observed visually or palpated and emphasize the degree of the problem. They play a major role, not only in assessment, but also in the follow-up of musculoskeletal problems. Hence, this chapter is presented to demonstrate how to formally document limb girths, limb lengths, chest excursion, and any other measurable physical findings, all of which must be tailored to the clinical setting. For example, the patient with a suspected L5 root lesion should have measurements made of calf circumference; a patient with a suspected meniscal tear should have measurements made of thigh girth **(Fig. 8-1)**. An examiner can easily forget to measure thigh girth in a patient with a knee complaint; therefore, this special chapter on measurements should serve as a reminder. Thigh girth should be taken at a fixed point such as the joint line rather than above an anatomical landmark of the knee such as the superior pole of the patella. Physicians debate whether this should be 4 or 10 inches above the joint line. Even chest excursion should be carefully measured, especially in a patient with spinal pain and a possible diagnosis of ankylosing spondylitis **(Fig. 8-2)**. A varus deformity, which can be seen when the patient is standing, can be measured by counting the number of fingers that can be positioned between the condyles **(Fig. 8-3)**.

Text continued on p. 242.

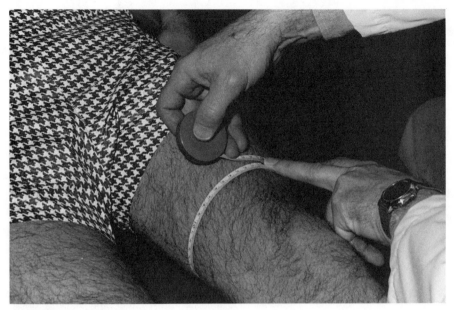

Figure 8-1.
Patients with suspected meniscal pathology should have their thigh girth measured. This can be performed a set distance above the knee joint and compared with the opposite side.

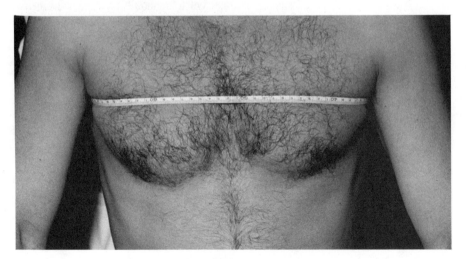

Figure 8-2.
Chest excursion should be carefully measured, especially in a patient with spinal pain and possible ankylosing spondylitis. Diminished chest excursion with large inhalation may indicate ankylosing spondylitis.

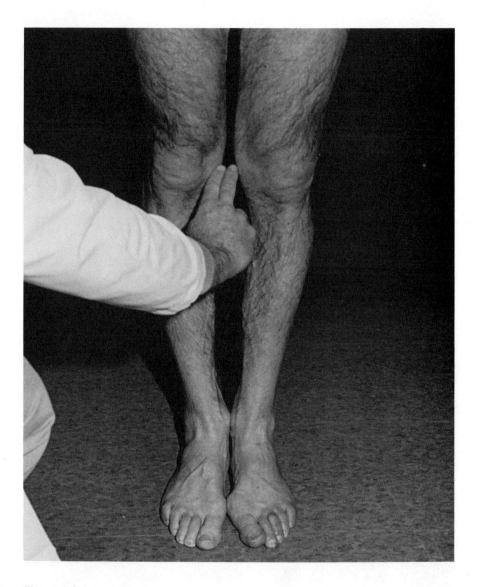

Figure 8-3.
A varus deformity is demonstrated, which can be objectively measured by counting the number of fingers that can be positioned between the femoral condyles.

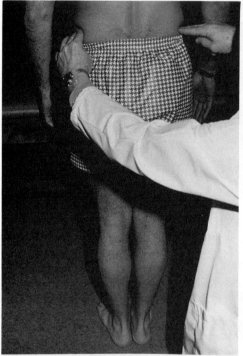

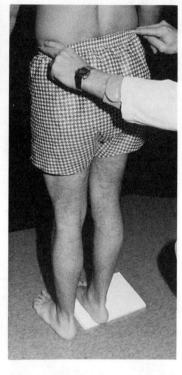

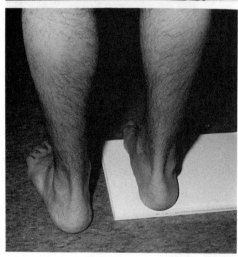

Figure 8-4.
A, A pelvic obliquity, which can be seen when the patient is standing, may suggest a discrepancy in leg lengths. B, Blocks can help equalize the pelvic obliquity when determining a discrepancy in leg lengths. Blocks can only be used, however, when no deformities of either the hip or the knee exist. C, The use of blocks to measure the height of the iliac crests is demonstrated.

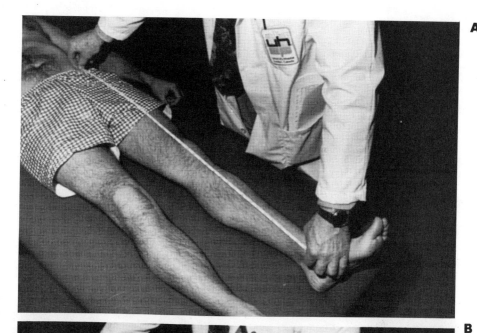

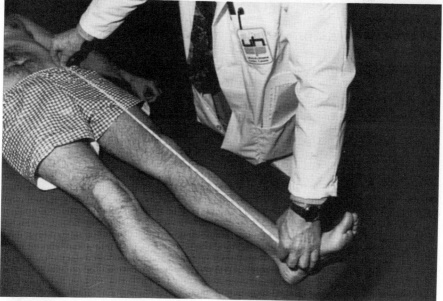

Figure 8-5.
A, A true leg length measurement taken from the anterior
superior iliac spine to the medial malleolus is demonstrated.
B, An apparent leg length measurement taken from a fixed
point in the midline such as a ziphi sternum to the medial
malleolus is demonstrated.

Assessment of limb lengths deserves special mention. Having determined whether any flexion deformities in the hip or knee or any other architectural deformities are present, measuring limb lengths is now appropriate. In the absence of flexion or other architectural deformities, the use of standing blocks to measure the level of the pelvis and the posterior iliac spine is reliable and accurate (Fig. 8-4).

Classically, *true limb length* is defined as a measurement from the anterior superior iliac spine to the medial malleolus (Fig. 8-5, A). If hip or knee deformities are present, however, the opposite extremity may require similar positioning to achieve as reliable a measure as possible. This is a particularly common concern with deformities of adduction and flexion of the hip. Alternatively, segmental measurements may be taken from the anterior superior iliac spine (ASIS) to a fixed point in the knee and then from the fixed point in the knee to the malleolus. The examiner should remember that *true* in this setting may be a misnomer in the measurement of true limb length.

Apparent limb length is measured from a fixed midline structure such as the sternum to the medial malleolus (Fig. 8-5, B). A difference between apparent and true limb length suggests the pathology is between the sternum and the anterior superior iliac spine, the most common of which probably would be a scoliosis.

Chapter

9   Vascularity

The significance of this aspect of physical examination cannot be overemphasized. In an acute injury, the most important determination on physical examination of the musculoskeletal system is documenting vascularity distal to the level of the lesion. Failure to document the vascular status of the extremity distal to a dislocated knee could prove disastrous. Vascularity is of such importance and encompasses such a wide spectrum of involvement that a separate section ensures its appropriate attention. Viability of an extremity, either acute or chronic, depends primarily on arterial perfusion. Only palpating for the presence of pulses may prove to be inadequate **(Fig. 9-1)**. In assessing vascularity, the examiner need not only consider pulses, but also skin temperature, color, and sensation. The old teaching adage consisting of the five P's of vascular impairment (pallor, pulselessness, pain, paresthesias, and poikilothermy) emphasizes the spectrum of vascular concern. This discussion of various conditions emphasizes the different physical examination features that may be noted.

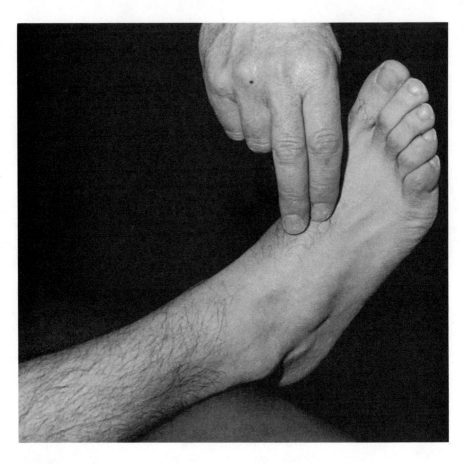

Figure 9-1.
Although palpation for the presence of pulses is important, performing that test alone when assessing viability of an extremity may be inadequate.

Acute Vascular Disruption

This may occur with a dislocated knee and a popliteal artery rupture or in a supracondylar fracture in a child with a brachial artery disruption. Assessment of pulses distal to the lesion is important, but the physician should also carefully note temperature, color, movement, sensation, and particularly capillary refill performed by blanching the nail bed and noting the rate of return to normal color from white to pink **(Fig. 9-2).** The absence of pulses in the upper extremity following a supracondylar fracture may be less ominous than the absence of pulses in the lower extremity following a dislocated knee because collateral circulation in the upper extremity is more abundant than in the lower. Viability is the primary concern. A cold, painful, immovable, numb, pulseless extremity with no capillary filling requires immediate attention and suggests significant vascular compromise, and possibly disruption. Recognizing significant vascular compromise early allows aggressive management and may lead to salvage rather than loss of a limb. Six hours' loss of blood supply is critical as to whether the limb may be saved.

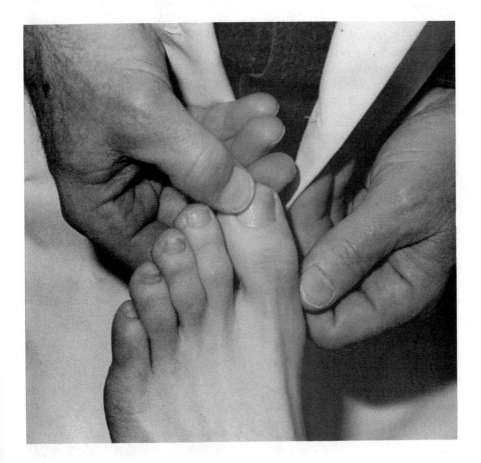

Figure 9-2.
One of the best determinants of viability of an extremity consists of assessing capillary refill. This is done by pressing the nail bed and noting the rate of return to normal color from white to pink upon release.

Compartment Syndromes

Compartment syndromes can develop following an acute injury, various forms of trauma, drug overdose, seizures, or vascular disruption. Frequently, the patient may complain of a disproportionate or inordinate amount of pain, not in keeping with the injury. Physical signs such as a swollen, tense compartment, loss of sensation and movement, and particularly increased pain on passive stretching of the part leads to a diagnosis. Passive stretching of the great toe into flexion causing significant pain suggests an anterior compartment syndrome in the lower extremity **(Fig. 9-3)**. Painful extension of fingers and wrist suggests a forearm flexor compartment syndrome in the upper extremity. Pulses are often present because the arterial pressure may be high enough to push blood through the larger vessels. Smaller vessel compromise resulting in muscle ischemia results from less diminished pressure. Some of

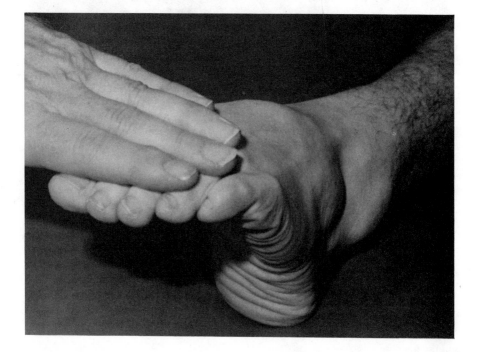

Figure 9-3.
Passive stretching of the great toe into flexion, which causes significant pain, suggests an anterior compartment syndrome following trauma or surgery in that area.

the physical signs of an acute vascular disruption may be present in addition to the important signs listed above of a compartment syndrome.

Following an acute ischemic injury, muscle contractures and deformities described as Volkmann's contracture may result if the acute ischemia is improperly treated.

Chronic Arterial Insufficiency

The patient with chronic arterial insufficiency presents with many different physical findings from the patient with an acute vascular insufficiency. For example, the patient who is a diabetic with small vessel disease may demonstrate temperature change, loss of sensation, skin changes such as loss of hair, shiny skin, or even ulceration. The palpable pulses are often diminished and capillary blush may be diminished. When operating on a patient with such problems, the physician must be aware of the potential consequences related to infection, and wound healing.

Venous Insufficiency

Venous insufficiency may lead to swelling, discoloration, induration, trophic changes, abnormal pigmentation, and even ulceration.

Thoracic Outlet

Specialized tests exist to diagnose thoracic outlet obstruction, which may be considered here or in a separate section on special tests. These consist of Adson's maneuver, the attention position, and a hyperabduction maneuver (**Fig. 7-18**). Each of these tests suggests pathological obstruction at different areas. Adson's maneuver consists of observing any diminution or elimination of the radial pulse by having the patient's arm abducted and extended, shoulders back, and looking in the opposite direction. The attention position consists of noting a diminution of the pulse by having the patient inhale maximally, thrusting the shoulders back. The hyperabduction test consists of noting any diminution or elimination of pulse by bringing the arm into the abducted position above 90 degrees. In each of these tests the two sides are compared. In some normal patients pulses may diminish with some of these tests.

See p. 232

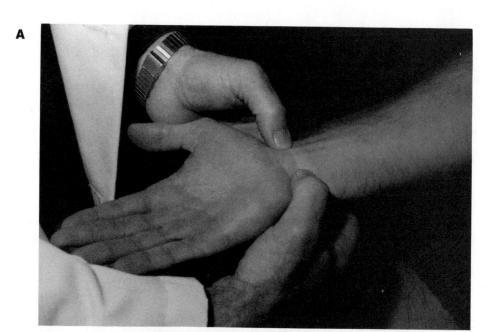

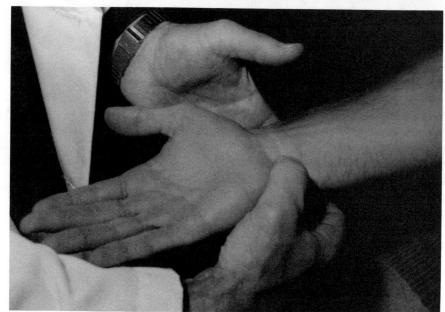

Figure 9-4.
A, B, Allen's test analyzes vascular competence of an
extremity. For example, in these illustrations, the examiner is
determining the contribution of the ulnar and the radial
arteries in supplying vascularity to the hand.

Perhaps the most reliable sign of thoracic outlet consists of reproducing the patient's upper extremity symptoms of paresthesias, discomfort, and heaviness when the hands are repetitively opened and closed with the arms in the forward elevated position **(see Fig. 7-19)**.

Allen's test can help distinguish which vessel is providing the predominant blood supply to a part. This test can distinguish contributions of blood supply to the hand from ulnar versus radial arteries **(Fig. 9-4, A, B)**.

Auscultation is not an integral part of the musculoskeletal examination, but under vascularity, listening to any areas where potential bruits may be present is important. This may occur over the femoral artery at the groin or following traumatic injuries in different areas of the body. Swellings that may be present, particularly if they are pulsatile or near a vascular supply, could represent a traumatic aneurysm and the presence of a bruit may aid in this diagnosis.

Chapter

10   Gait Analysis

During the initial impression and before the formal physical examination, the physician should have formulated an opinion regarding the patient's ambulation and gait. Many gait patterns are obvious as they relate to different pathologies and can be accurately assessed upon first visual observation. Often, the patient who has bilateral dysplasia of the hip walks with an obvious bilateral Trendelenburg gait. The patient who has an L5 root neurological lesion in the lower extremity may present with a drop foot and a classical inability to dorsiflex the ankle, with a resounding slap as the patient walks across the floor. Similarly, the patient who has diabetic tabes dorsalis or some other form of posterior column disease presents with an ataxic shuffling gait. An accurate gait analysis can be established after assessing deformities, contractures, limb lengths, and neurological function. Until these factors have been determined, accurately assessing the gait pattern could prove difficult. This formal determination can reasonably be left until the end of the examination.

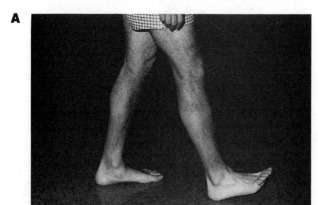

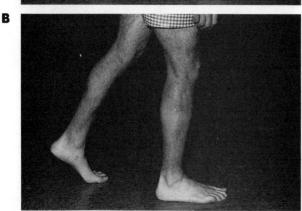

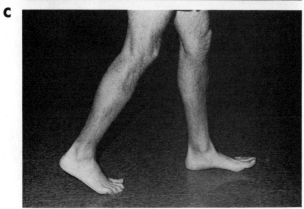

Figure 10-1.
A, Gait analysis consists of heel-strike, demonstrated here on the right foot. B, In gait analysis following heel-strike, patients go into mid-stance, demonstrated here on the right foot. C, Following midstance, patients then go into toe-off, demonstrated here on the right foot.

Gait analysis observing the stance and swing phases notes the rhythm, cadence, timing, and agility with which these phases are performed. For example, a patient with an antalgic gait has an abreviated stance phase. The stance phase consists of heel-strike **(Fig. 10-1, A)** midstance **(Fig. 10-1, B)**, and toe-off **(Fig. 10-1, C)**. The swing phase consists of acceleration, midswing, and deceleration **(Fig. 10-2)**. An additional analysis is made relative to the various muscle actions and joint movements as the patient walks. The use of walking aids or influence of artificial limbs must be taken into consideration. A broad classification of gait must be developed, which might be based on underlying cause such as neurological, muscular, architectural, or some descriptive term such as *Trendelenburg*. Unfortunately, a practical or simple classification of gait abnormalities is not readily available.

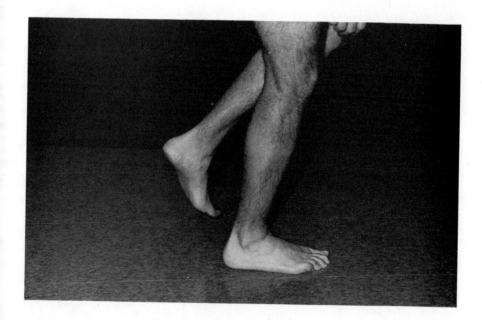

Figure 10-2.
While examining the right lower extremity for heel-strike, midstance, and toe-off, the opposite extremity goes through swing phases of acceleration, midswing, and deceleration.

Chapter

11

General Assessment

All patients should be considered for a general assessment, which may include cardiorespiratory, abdominal, genitourinary, and occasionally rectal examination. Without a complete physical examination, the physician might fail to detect systemic disease, which may cause or relate to a specific musculoskeletal complaint. For example, detection of an enlarged, hard prostate might suggest that a patient's hip pain may be caused by metastatic prostatic carcinoma. Bypassing a rectal exam in patients who have had either an acute or long-standing spinal cord injury with neurological compromise would result in an incomplete examination. A patient's future bladder function following an acute spinal cord injury may well depend upon the findings on a rectal examination. This might dictate the level and method of eventual neurological return relating to bladder function. Patients who have aortic stenosis associated with Marfan's syndrome may present with multidirectional instability of the shoulder. Patients with blue sclera may have an associated diagnosis of osteogenesis imperfecta.

Patients with musculoskeletal complaints occasionally require surgery and their suitability for surgery must be determined. Even young patients undergoing outpatient knee arthroscopy should not only have an examination of the musculoskeletal system, but also a general examination including the cardiovascular and respiratory systems to ensure fitness for surgery. A careful physical examination will often detect problems such as an obvious heart murmur or previous respiratory complications associated with asthma and should be done before the patient undergoes surgery.

An elderly patient with a hip fracture requiring surgery must be given a thorough general examination to ensure fitness for surgery. If problems exist, they should be brought under control or at least brought into the best shape possible before the surgery. Based on physical examination, such patients may be poor candidates for surgery, and knowing the expectations and risks is necessary. Often elderly patients are distressed with heart or respiratory difficulties, and these features are evident after a simple assessment.

Patients acutely injured, especially in motor vehicle accidents, warrant a thorough assessment related to the ABC's of trauma management to rule out other more life-threatening injuries. This requires documentation of the patient's general status before proceeding to more specific musculoskeletal problems.

Patients who are comatose following an accident, especially one involving a motor vehicle, must have examination of the cervical spine and pelvis as well as appropriate ancillary investigations in those areas.

Chapter

12   Special Considerations

Special considerations and circumstances dictate a modified approach to physical examination. In newborns, the neurological examination must be done largely by observation and some form of stimulus testing. In the child who presents with a very painful extremity, the apprehension may be so significant that examination of that part should be left to the very end of the process. In the patient who presents in a coma following a motor vehicle accident, physical examination may be rapidly assimilated while treatment is instituted. Stimuli of a painful nature may be the only way to determine aspects such as level of consciousness and certain areas of pathology such as fractures.

Special considerations concerning examination of the cervical, thoracic, and lumbar spine, and the hand also exist. These anatomical areas are unique, but nevertheless require examination that fits with the general format described herein. The spine and the hand may require extra experience with attention to certain details. Nevertheless, adhering to the principles previously outlined will allow the physician to formulate the appropriate diagnosis. A brief description of the spinal examination demonstrates how it fits into the same format.

Cervical Spine

In the cervical spine, the emphasis is on the position of the head; range of motion of the neck; and areas of localized tenderness with specialized attention to a neurological examination of the upper extremities and, occasionally, upper motor neuron signs in the lower extremities.

Inspection

Patients with cervical spine problems may present with attitude abnormalities such as typical torticollis or a cock robin position. Likewise, those with cervical instability sometimes present with their neck thrust forward. Patients with ankylosing spondylitis may have a lordotic or kyphotic deformity of the cervical spine, or kyphosis lower down in the thoracic spine with compensatory lordosis in the cervical spine. The paravertebral spinal muscles may appear hypertrophied due to spasticity and pain. This is more meaningful if enlargement occurs only on one side.

Palpation of the Cervical Spine

Palpation of the midline cervical structures may reveal tenderness over the spinous processes. Such tenderness is almost always present in patients with degenerative disk disease. Palpating along the paracervical musculature may reveal areas of localized point tenderness or generalized tenderness caused by muscle spasm.

Range of Motion

Range of motion of the cervical spine consists of flexion and extension, lateral flexion (tilt), and rotation (see Figs. 4-18, 4-19, 4-21, 4-22 on pp 90, 91, 95). These methods of documentation have been previously described. Assessment of stability of the cervical spine is not very significant, but the examiner might look for the thrust forward position of the cervical spine.

Neurological Examination

When examining the cervical spine, an appropriate motor, sensory, and reflex assessment of both upper extremities must be performed. The physician must keep in mind both the root innervation from C5 to T1, as well as the peripheral nerve innervation of the upper extremities when considering neurological examination.

Abduction of the shoulders, C5; flexion of the elbows, C6; extension of the elbows and wrists, C7; and abduction of the index finger, C8; and of the baby finger, T1 is a simple cursory motor root neurological examination of the upper extremities. A simple sensory examination considers the roots of C5 over the lateral deltoid, C6; palmar tip of thumb or index finger, C7; palmar tip of the long fingers, C8; palmar aspect of the distal baby finger, and the medial aspect of the upper arm, T1 (see Table

5-1). Two-point discrimination following peripheral nerve injuries is often meaningful.

Reflex examination consists of biceps reflex and brachioradiales reflex, C6; triceps reflex, C7; and profundus reflex of the fingers, C8 (see Table 5-1).

Special Tests

Special tests of the cervical spine consist of compression (see Fig. 7-6, A) and distraction (Fig. 7-6, B), as well as Spurling's test (see Fig. 7-6, C). (See Fig. 7-6, A-C on p 221.)

Thoracic Spine

Assessing the thoracic spine often focuses on malalignment abnormalities such as scoliosis that are associated with rib humps, along with kyphosis and lordosis. Considerable specialized testing exists in examining for scoliosis, e.g., documenting whether the curve is compensated. Having established a diagnosis of scoliosis, referring the patient to a pediatric orthopedic surgeon with an interest in the care of such problems is important. The reader should refer to standard pediatric texts for a detailed description of physical examinations for patients with scoliosis.

Lumbar Spine

Examination of the lumbar spine commonly required in patients who present with back pain requires elaboration. Initially, the patient is examined standing and observed walking. Provocative testing, noting subtle weakness, can be performed with these activities (Fig. 12-1). The bulk of the neurological examination may be performed in the sitting position. Straight leg raising is assessed in the supine position, while further neurological testing is performed. The appropriate sciatic and femoral stretch tests are performed supine. As the patient walks, the examiner must analyze the gait, noting whether any neurological deficiencies such as a drop foot are present. Provocative walking on toes and heels may elicit any weakness of plantar or dorsiflexion. Further provocative testing by having the patient go up and down on toes and up and down on the flexed knee elicits any plantar flexion or quadriceps weakness suggestive of root involvement (Fig. 12-1).

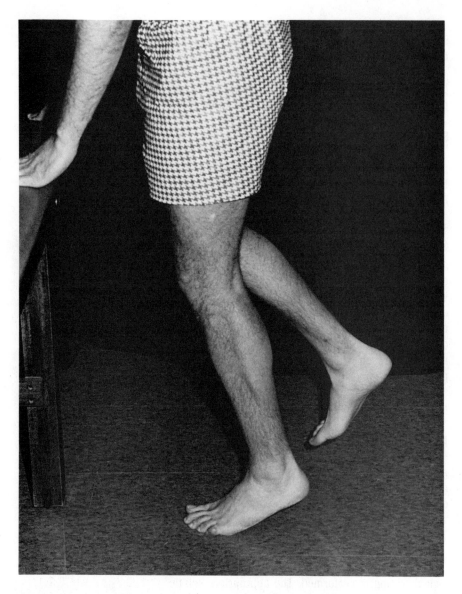

Figure 12-1.
Provocative testing for neurological weakness is performed
when examining the lumbar spine. This patient demonstrates
plantar flexion strength by going up and down on the toes
several times to elicit any weakness. This patient could also
perform up and down knee flexion, looking for quadriceps
weakness if it is present.

In the standing position, any malalignment and attitude abnormalities, pelvic obliquity, or presence of a Trendelenburg sign are noted (see Fig. 7-5 on p 219). Cursory assessment of leg lengths are made (see Fig. 8-4, A on p 240). Range of motion of the lumbar spine is important (see Figs. 4-17, 4-19, 4-43, 4-44 on pp 89, 91, 114, 115). Tenderness along the posterior lumbar spine or adjacent musculature is often present with low back pain (Fig. 12-2).

Office practitioners often find sitting on a stool facing the patient an appropriate way to perform a neurologi-

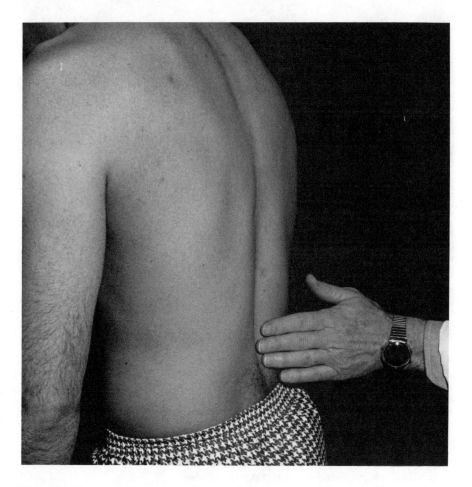

Figure 12-2.
Tenderness over the posterior lumbar spine and/or of the paralumbar musculature is often present with low back pain.

cal examination. In this position, performing motor, sensory, and reflex assessment and determining root involvement is easy.

Straight leg raising can be done in the sitting position **(Fig. 12-3)**, although the patient's back must be held forward. This is a helpful test when looking for a malingerer who has negative straight leg raising sitting

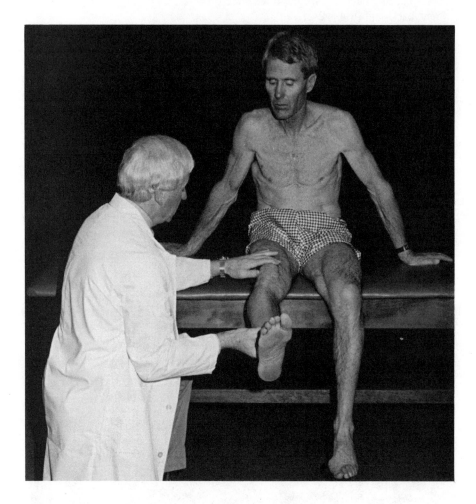

Figure 12-3.
Straight leg raising can be demonstrated in the sitting position. The examiner should ensure that the patient's back is held forward. This test is helpful in checking for a malingerer who has negative straight leg raising sitting and positive straight leg raising supine.

and positive straight leg raising supine.

In the supine position, further neurological testing can be done along with Lasègue's sign, or straight leg raising in which pain is elicited and referred to the distribution of the posterior thigh or sciatic nerve **(Fig. 12-4).** This represents a positive Lasègue's sign; the second component of straight leg raising or Lasègue's

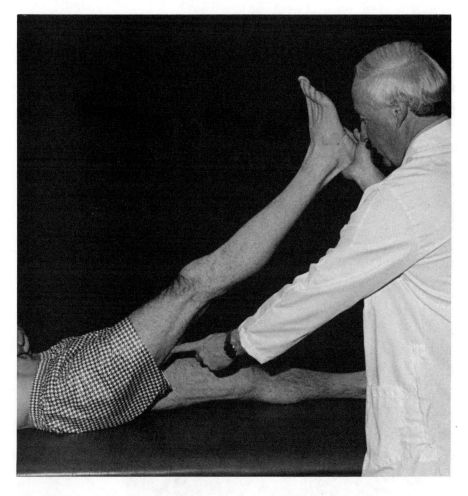

Figure 12-4.
Classical straight leg raising or Lasègue's sign in which pain is elicited and referred to the distribution of the sciatic nerve or the posterior thigh is shown. The second component of straight leg raising or Lasègue's sign consists of flexing the knee and hip to eliminate the pain.

sign consists of flexing the knee and hip to eliminate the pain. Straight leg raising may be augmented with forcible dorsiflexion of the ankle **(Fig. 12-5)**. Bowstringing is performed with the foot on the examiner's shoulder while sitting on the examining table **(Fig. 12-6)**. The knee is held in the extended position that just produces sciatic irritation down the posterior thigh, and that pain is then augmented with direct pressure over the popliteal fossa and tibial nerve.

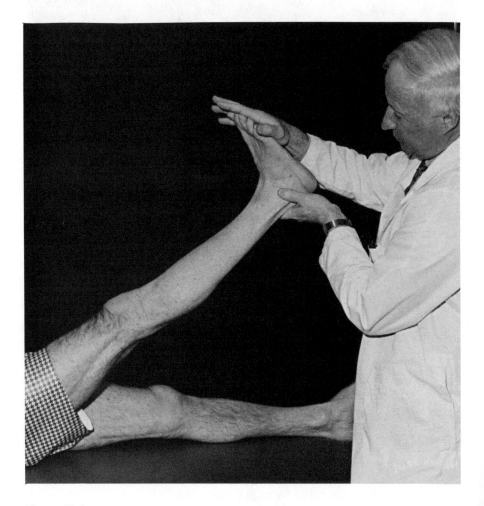

Figure 12-5.
Straight leg raising or Lasègue's sign may be augmented by forcibly dorsiflexing the ankle, increasing the pain in the distribution of the sciatic nerve.

Pushing on the hamstrings in this position indicates whether hamstring tightness is causing the pain. The femoral stretch test is performed prone with the knee flexed 90 degrees by lifting the leg toward the ceiling, eliciting pain in the distribution of the femoral nerve or in the anterior thigh (**Fig. 12-7**).

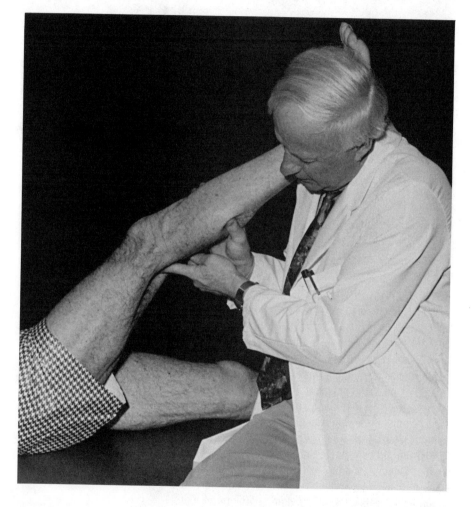

Figure 12-6.
Bowstringing is performed with the foot on the examiner's shoulder, backing off slightly from a positive straight leg raising test, and pushing over the posterior tibial nerve and the popliteal fossa. Eliciting pain radiating to the posterior thigh is a positive bowstring.

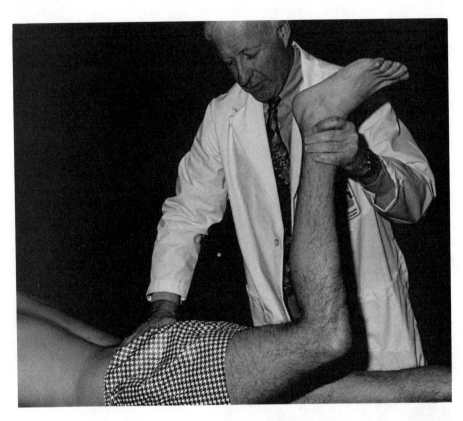

Figure 12-7.

The femoral stretch test, which is indicative of a femoral nerve irritation, is performed prone with the knee flexed 90 degrees by lifting the leg upward. Pain referred to the anterior thigh is a positive femoral stretch test.

The common roots assessed in such an examination are L2, L3, L4, L5, and S1 and S2 (see Table 5-5). L2 sensory diminution is in the anterior groin area with motor weakness of adduction of the hip. L3 sensory diminution is in the upper anterior thigh with weakness of hip flexion. L4 consists of diminution of response to pinprick over the distal anterior thigh with weakness of knee extension or quadriceps function. A diminished knee jerk with L4 lesions is also found. L5 consists of diminution in response to pinprick over the distal medial lower extremity, as well as along the lateral border of the foot with weakness of ankle dorsiflex. Some report this as more predominantly an L4 motor response. L5 diminution is exhibited by dullness to pinprick in the web space. S1 sensory loss is along the sole of the foot medially and weakness of plantar flexion of the ankle, along with a diminished ankle jerk. These guidelines can be followed but may vary among textbooks.

Chapter

13

Specialized Testing of the Hand

Because of the specialized function of the hand and the many joints involved, the examination becomes seemingly subspecialized, and comprehensive examination of a hand takes much longer compared with that, say, of the knee. Specialized tests such as assessing intrinsic contractures with Bunnell's test, describing the characteristic deformities of rheumatoid arthritis (**Fig. 13-1**), or specific functional testing of the hand may require particular focus. The principles and format of this examination are the same, even though the physician must concentrate on more parts and occasionally perform more specialized tests.

Inspection and cursory assessment of the hand consists of examining for any deformities, posture attitude, muscle wasting, swelling, and discoloration as is done for any other part. Examination of the nails may also reveal abnormalities. By palpation, aspects such as tenderness, swelling, and synovial crepitus may be noted.

Range of motion analyzes the wrist, the metacarpophalangeal and interphalangeal joints of the fingers, and the joints of the thumb. The ranges are documented in degrees and any contractures are documented. Strength testing is conducted, considering root and peripheral nerve innervation, and helps assess function about the joints of the hand. This is followed by comprehensive motor, sensory, and neurological examination of the hand.

Special testing of the hand may consist of the following:

1. Allen's test to analyze vascular competence **(Fig. 13-1, A, B)**

2. Tinel's sign at the wrist, suggesting median nerve compression **(Fig. 13-2)**

3. Phalen's test, suggesting median nerve compression **(Fig. 13-3)**

4. Finkelstein's test, suggesting tendinitis of thumb abductors **(Fig. 13-4)**

5. Bunnell's test

Deformities of the hand, particularly in the patient with rheumatoid arthritis or in the patient post trauma, may be obvious **(Fig. 13-5)**. These include, but are not limited to, mallet fingers with fixed flexion of the distal interphalangeal joint, boutonniére deformity with hyperextension of the proximal interphalangeal joint, and flexion of the distal interphalangeal joint, swan neck deformities, and ulnar drift.

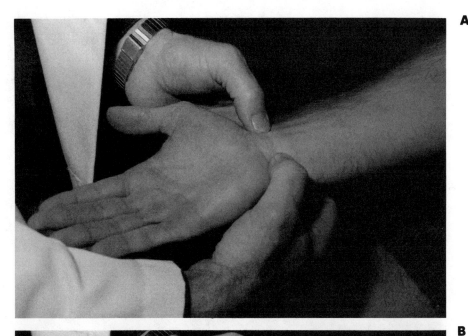

A

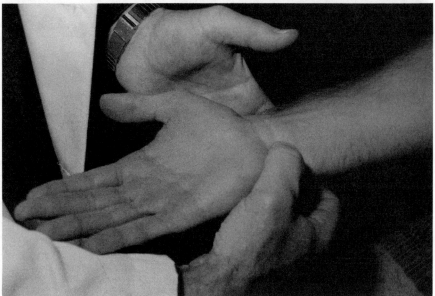

B

Figure 13-1.

A, B, Allen's test analyzes vascular competence of an extremity. For example, in these illustrations, the examiner is determining the contribution of the ulnar and the radial arteries in supplying vascularity to the hand.

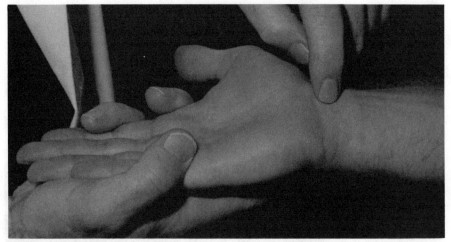

Figure 13-2.
Tinel's test, performed at the wrist, may produce paresthesias
and pain in the distribution of the median nerve.

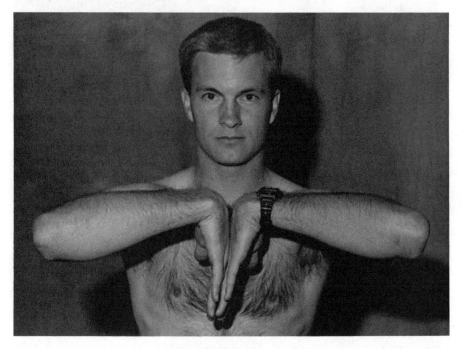

Figure 13-3.
Phalen's test has the patient forcibly flexing the wrists
together, reproducing pain and paresthesias in the distribution of the median nerve, suggestive of a carpal tunnel
syndrome.

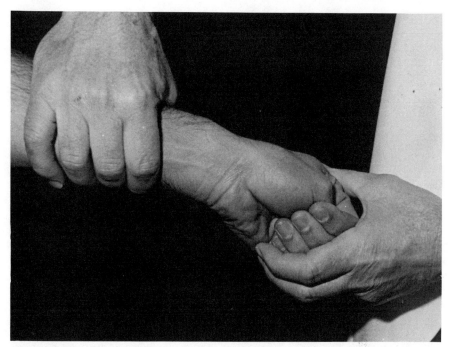

Figure 13-4.
Finkelstein's test suggests tendinitis of the thumb abductors, and is performed by forcing the flexed and adducted thumb across the palm, stretching the tendons and causing pain.

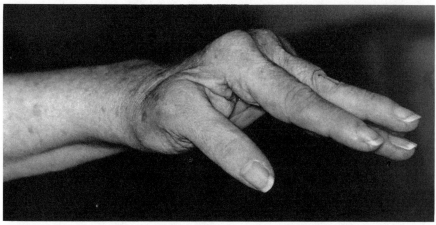

Figure 13-5.
Specialized considerations in the hand include the deformities that occur with rheumatoid arthritis.

Chapter

14   Conclusion

Through this format the physician has been encouraged to examine not only the site of primary focus, but also the joint above and below the involved part. During the examination, physicians also have been urged to integrate other features of physical examination in other parts of the body that may prove relevant. Although this format has been presented in a segmented manner, many of the segments actually overlap and are performed simultaneously. Experience and repetition allows physicians to be more effective in developing this aspect of the "art" of examination.

With a knowledge of the anatomy and the pathology and having assimilated the above information, applying the principles of common things being common to arrive at the most likely diagnosis is now appropriate. The diagnosis may only be provisional, in which case the physician should now proceed to appropriate investigative techniques, such as radiological assessment laboratory investigations and other specialized procedures.

Once the initial data base has been established and all pertinent problems are listed, the examiner may record impression(s) and prepare a preliminary or provisional diagnosis with accompanying differential diagnoses given in order of priority. Confirmation of the diagnosis may require a variety of laboratory and roentgenographic tests. The examiner needs to decide if other data are needed to screen for a missed illness and what other data would be helpful in identifying or managing a disease entity already described.

Once diagnostic studies (history, physical examination, and laboratory data) have defined the problem, treatment may be instituted. The patient should be included in the management process.

Finally, appropriate progress notes should document the outcome of the problem. The notes should include subjective and objective information, such as pertinent laboratory data. They should also state the examiner's analysis of the information and any treatment changes and the reasons for the change.

Presentation of the Patient

Having completed the history and physical examination, the physician should endeavor to present the findings on history in an orderly, clear fashion and that the physical signs, either verbally or clinically, are demonstrated in the appropriate manner. (The manner in which to present the history has already been discussed.)

While presenting a clinical summary to colleagues, the physician must convey in a concise fashion the chief complaint of the patient as perceived by the patient, while providing a clear impression of the degree of disability or pain as it has evolved from its date of inception to the present, noting its progress over time and the influence of any treatment. History and physical examination should be presented and written in an organized fashion, illustrating all pertinent positive, and sometimes even negative, findings. A concise logical progression will ease presentation and convey greater clinical acumen. For example, in verbal presentation, the summary would begin, "This 69-year-old male farmer presents with a chief complaint of hip pain. His history dates back seven years when he fell from the barn roof." The pertinent relevant clinical findings are based on inspection, palpation, range of motion, and other aspects of the previously described format.

In presenting the physical examination findings, emphasizing the positive features, commenting upon negative features only if relevant to exclude a considered diagnosis, is appropriate. When demonstrating the physical examination findings at the bedside or to colleagues, the physician should make the signs and tests visible, which obviously depends upon their perspective. At the bedside, when presenting physical signs to another individual, that individual can then easily position himself so not to compromise the physical examination. On the other hand, when presenting physical examination signs to a large group of students, particularly in an auditorium, the audience must be allowed to visualize the examination, which may mean a compromise on the examiner's part. For example, in demonstrating range of motion of the right hip, the right hip should be clearly adjacent to the audience and the examiner on the opposite side (i.e., the left side of the patient) so as not to obstruct the view of the audience.

Discussion with the Patient

At the completion of the history and physical examination the physician must discuss all the relevant issues with the patient, including findings, diagnosis, prognosis, and a suggested treatment plan if applicable at this time. Further investigative procedures may be required to establish the diagnosis, which may allow only an abbreviated guess of what might be the problem. Physicians are frequently guilty of not spending enough time with patients explaining to them what is involved, what the diagnosis is, what the treatment plan involves, and what the future holds. Nothing is more frustrating to a patient than to feel, upon leaving the doctor, that he has neither had the appropriate time nor been told the ramifications of the situation. Quite often patients state that the physician did not perform a thorough exam or offer a diagnosis after the exam. The physician needs time and patience, which vary with the depth of knowledge and appreciation of the patient. The physician must explain to the patient, as best as can be done, what the future holds, given the patient's particular situation. If patients can be assured the problem is a self-limiting disease that will improve with appropriate treatment, they are much more content than facing the unknown. On the other hand, if the situation is progressive, that, too, requires clarification.

Physicians frequently recommend surgery, and in such circumstances, they are compelled to explain the pros and cons and ramifications of the surgery, the expectation and outcome of the disease process with and without surgery, and the possible complications material to that procedure. Then, too, many of these same issues need to be discussed when surgery is not contemplated. This is an aspect of an informed consent that all physicians have a responsibility to provide.

Physicians are often criticized for not listening to patients. Patients must be given an opportunity to express their opinions both during the course of the initial questioning and/or at the examination's end, with a specific question to patients regarding any questions they have, allowing them to express their feelings. Answering all the questions that patients have about the problem greatly allays their apprehension and fear, thereby providing confidence in their physicians.

Finally, after the physician has discussed the diagnosis and recommended treatment program, the patient should be asked pointed questions, such as

Do you understand?
Do you have any questions?
Is this treatment plan acceptable to you?

Frequently, patients do not express their feelings without being asked specific questions.

Summary

In summary, the goal of the examination is to obtain a diagnosis if possible or to obtain enough pertinent information to direct further evaluation.

When presenting the case to others, clarity is important, and the audience and/or colleagues should have a clear idea of the patient from the presentation of the history in terms of degree of problem and from the positive physical findings in terms of our musculoskeletal assessment. Useless information should be eliminated from the presentation. Both the examiner and colleagues should form an opinion on the patient's condition based on the presentations of history and physical examination. Finally, objective documentation is critical, both for medical charting and for presentation to colleagues.

Suggested Reading

1. American Academy of Orthopaedic Surgeons: *Joint motion: Methods of measuring and recording,* Illinois, 1965, AAOS.
2. Bates, B: *A guide to physical examination,* ed 3, Philadelphia, 1983, JB Lippincott, pp. 340–355.
3. Cave EF, Roberts SM: A method for measuring and recording joint function. *J Bone Joint Surg* 34:455, 1936.
4. Delp MH, Mainning RT: *Major's physical diagnosis,* ed 8, Philadelphia, 1975, WB Saunders, pp. 637–699.
5. Hawkins RJ, Murnaghan JP: *The shoulder in adult orthopaedics.* In RL Cruess, WRJ Rennie, editors: New York, 1984, Churchill Livingstone, pp. 949–959.
6. Hawkins RJ: Examination of the shoulder. *J Orthop* 6(10):1270–1278, 1983.
7. Post ME: *Physical examination of the musculoskeletal system.* Chicago/London, 1986, Yearbook Medical Publishers.

Index*

---

*A t after the page number indicates a table.
An f indicates a figure.

B

Babinski reflex, 151
Babinski response, positive, 144f
Back pain, 259–261
Biceps brachii muscle
  testing of, 153t, 156t
Biceps femoris, testing of, 165t
Biceps muscle
  reflex of, 147f, 159
  root levels of, 152t
  ruptured, 53f, 57
  strength testing of, 134f
Biceps tendon, tenderness of, 67f
Bilateral comparison, 29
Bladder assessment, 168
Blood loss, 245
Body habitus, 34
Bone damage, 18
Bony swelling, 62
Boutonniére deformity, 268
Bowel function, 168
Bowstringing, 265f
Brachial plexus lesion, deformity with, 55
Brachialis testing, 153t
Brachioradialis
  reflex of, 160
  testing of, 153t
Bruising, 48
Bunion, malalignment with, 48
Bunnell's test, 268

C

C7 root lesion, 56–57
Café au lait spot, 57
Capillary filling assessment, 245
Capital femoral epiphysis, 129f
  slipped, 126
Capsulitis, adhesive, 16, 102
Carpal tunnel syndrome, 143–145, 229, 270f
  testing for, 230f
Carpometacarpal joint motion, 112
Catching, 17
Cellulitis, 62
Cervical spine
  extension of, 91f
  flexion distances in, 87
  inspection of, 257–258
  instability, areas of pathology in, 28
  lateral flexion of, 95f
  neurologic assessment of, 147–148, 258–259

palpation of, 258
physical examination for, 25–26
range of motion of, 258
rotation of, 95f
special considerations for, 257–259
special tests for, 220, 221f, 259
suspected fracture of, 148
Chest excursion, 238f
  measurement of, 237
Chief complaint, 1–2, 4–5
  areas of, 27–28
  current status of, 9
  degree of pain or disability with, 13–14
  events surrounding, 7
  instability as, 14–16
  obtaining history of, 7–21
  pain as, 10–13
  progression of, 8–9
  symptoms as, 16–18
Chin, flexion of, 90f
Clavicular reflex, 160
Clinical course, 8
Clinical instability testing, 169–179
Clinical setting, 4
Clinical summary, 274–275
Clonus, sustained, 143f
Cock robin position, 257
Collagen tissue deficiency, 52, 169
Color, inspection of, 48
Comatose patient, 256
Compartment syndromes, 246–247
Compression test, 259
Contractures, 122–126
Contusion, 148
Coracobrachialis muscle testing, 156t
Coronal plane, 103
  abduction in, 105f
  elevation in, 81f
Crank test, 176–177f, 186
Crepitus, 130–132
  in knee instability, 204–205
  of snapping scapula, 227
Crossed arm abduction, 225f
Cubitus valgus, 45
Current illness
  obtaining history of, 7–21
  onset of, 7–8
Cystic swelling, 48

D

Data base, 273
Deformities
  with acute injury, 18

Joints—cont'd
deformities of
motion with, 122–126
examination of, 30–31
excessive flexibility of, 170f
fluid in, 62
lining irritation, swelling with, 17
motion of
abnormal, 122
active vs. passive, 122
degrees of, 84–86
stability assessment of, 169–214
stiffness as chief complaint, 16
swelling of, 48–52

K

Keegan's map, 157
Keloid, 52
Klumpke's palsy, 55
Knee
crepitus of, 130, 131f
dislocated, ecchymosis of, 48
excessive recurvatum of, 190f, 202
flexion assessment of, 28f
flexion of, 118f
degrees of, 85
flexion rotation test of, 194f
hyperextension of, 190f
instability of, 14–15, 170, 171f
patellar, 175, 176f
ligamentous instability testing of, 192
locked, 126
medial collateral ligament instability of,
171f
medial instability of, 170
medial opening of, 172–173
meniscal tear in, 55–56
palpating for tenderness of, 68f
motion of, 117
pain in, 206–207
physical examination for, 25–26
passive extension of, 74f
postoperative flexion deformity of, 83f
range of motion of, 132f, 194–198
septic, 43f
special tests for, 234–236
stability assessment of, 174–175,
189–207
swelling at, 48–49, 49–51
testing fluid on, 49, 51f, 62
twisting injury to, 49–52
varus and valgus of, 46f

Kyphosis
definition of, 94t
diagnosis of, 259
Kyphotic deformity, 258

L

L4 motor response, 266
L5 root lesion, 57
Lachman maneuver, reverse, 197f, 203
Lachman test, 192f, 194f, 199
positive, 200f
reverse, 202–203
Lasègue's sign, 263–264
Latissimus dorsi testing, 155t
Laxity
assessment of, 169–214
patient demonstration of, 178
Leg; see Lower extremities
Leg length measurement, 241f
Lhermitte's sign, 222
Lifestyle, pain and, 13
Lift-off test, 226f, 227
Limbs; see also Lower extremities; Upper
extremities
absent, 52
length
apparent, 242
assessment of, 241f, 242
true, 242
Limp, 35
Linear pain scale analogue, 13
Listening, 275–276
to patient's complaint, 3
Litigation, with acute injury, 18
Load and shift test, 182, 183f
Locking, 17
Lordosis
definition of, 94t
of thoracic spine, 259
Lordotic deformity, 258
Losee maneuver, 193f, 202
Lower extremities
absence of pulses in, 245
anterior compartment syndrome in, 246
muscle testing chart for, 164–166t
neurologic examination of, 168
neurologic root levels in, 167t
peripheral nerve assessment of, 167t
Lumbar spine
extension of, 90–93
flexion of, 89f
lateral flexion of, 114f

Neurologic examination—cont'd
of lumbar spine, 259–260, 262–265
modification of, 141–143
with muscle wasting, 56
in physical examination format, 30–31
of upper limbs, 152–167
Neurologic pathology, paresthesias with, 18
Neurologic root levels, 152t, 258
of lower extremities, 167t
Neurologic strength testing, 132f, 133
Neurologic tests, special, 233
Neuropathy, 231f
Nevus discoloration, 57
Numbness, 143–145

O

Ober's test, 234
Obturator nerve assessment, 167t
Onset, 7–8
Opponens digiti quinti testing, 154t
Opponens pollicis testing, 154t
Ortolani's sign, 209–210, 233–234
Barlow's modification of, 211f, 233–234
Osmond-Clarke test, 204, 234
modification of, 205f
Osteoarthritis
crepitus with, 132
muscle wasting with, 56
tests for, 234
Osteochondroma, 63
Osteogenesis imperfecta, 255
Osteomyelitis, swelling with, 48–49
Osteophyte formation, 62

P

Pain
with active elevation, 127f
with active motion, 128f
activity restriction with, 12
with acute injury, 18
attitude and, 44
back, 259–261
as chief complaint, 10–13
in compartment syndromes, 246
degree of, 13–14
elimination of with support, 128f
intensity of, 13
lifestyle and personality factors in, 13
from meniscal vs. ligamentous
pathology, 234, 235f
with motion, 126

in muscle testing, 136, 137f, 140
night, 11–12
origin of, 11
quality of, 11
with resisted dorsiflexion of wrist, 228
shoulder, palpation for, 68–69
with stressed external rotation, 129f
treatment effects on, 12
Painful arc, 215, 218f
with shoulder impingement, 223, 224f
Palmar flexion, 109f
Palmar interossei testing, 154t
Palpation, 61–69
of cervical spine, 258
for pulses, 244f
Paravertebral spinal muscle hypertrophy, 258
Paresthesia
as chief complaint, 18
in thoracic outlet syndrome, 249
at wrist, 270f
Parkinsonism, abnormal movement rhythm
with, 129
Passive motion, 73f
definition of, 71
in elderly, 122, 123f
joint, 122
testing of, 73–82
Patella
compression of, 236f
crepitus of, 130, 131f
dislocated, 52
height of, 205–206
instability of, 175, 176f
laxity assessment of, 203–204
stability assessment of, 203–207
Patellar ballottement, 52f, 62
Patellar tap, 62
Patellar tendon assessment, 206f
Patellofemoral instability, 203–207
Pathology, primary areas of, 27–28
Patient
age of, 1–2
discussion with, 275–276
listening to, 275–276
presentation of, 274–275
Patient positioning, 40
during inspection, 41, 42–44
Pectoralis major testing, 156t
Pectoralis minor testing, 156t
Pectoralis reflex, 160
Pelvic obliquity, 240f
Peripheral nerve
assessment

Varus, 118, 121f
  definition of, 94t
  deformity, 45
    measurement of, 237, 239f
  instability
    eliciting of, 191f
    knee, 198–200
  knee, 46f
  stress, at elbow, 208–209
Vascular competence, 268, 269f
Vascular disruption
  acute, 244–245
  compartment syndromes with, 246
  physical signs of, 247
Vascular impairment, five P's of, 243
Vascular viability, 245
Vascularity assessment, 49f, 243–249
Venous insufficiency, 247
Volkmann's contracture, 247